Between the Hips

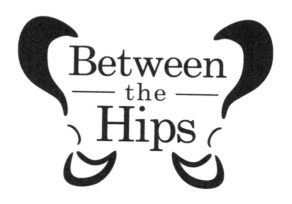

A Practical Guide for Women

Dr. Megan Rorabeck, DPT, WCS

To all of the strong women out there—which is every woman out there—especially my grandmothers, Mary Lou and Louise. I love you.

CONTENTS

ACKNOWLEDGMENTS

It would be a disservice if I did not take this opportunity to thank all of the people in my life who've helped make not only this book, but also my career as a physical therapist possible.

First, I must thank my husband, Brian. Words will never be able to express how grateful I am for you. Despite my manic tendencies at times with my dreams, desires, and "projects," you never fail to support and encourage me.

To my parents, Jeff and Michele Neitzel, thank you for valuing my education and making it possible for me to attend school to become a Doctor of Physical Therapy. Thank you for your endless encouragement, love, and support in my endeavors.

To my sister, Paige Woggon, thank you for always believing in me as your big sister. From the days you called me "Mema" because "Megan" was too hard, until now and forever, I promise to always be your best friend.

To my mother-in-law, Loretta Rorabeck, and my grandmothers, Elizabeth Oswald, Kay Rorabeck, Louise Vinz, and Mary Lou Neitzel, thank you for being a light of kindness, strength, hope, wisdom, encouragement, and love in my life.

To my physical therapy colleges and professors and Carroll University and my writing and physical therapy mentors (there are too many to name, but you know who you are), thank you for helping pave the way, teaching me all you know, being patient with me, and giving your encouragement to be the best physical therapist I can possibly be.

To my editor, Renee Nicholls; book designer, Claire MacMaster; and cover designer, Stacy Harmeling; thank you for your tireless efforts to help make this book possible. Teamwork really does make the dream work!

Lastly, and perhaps most importantly, I must thank my patients. Their courage, relentless search for answers and solutions, and trust in me as their physical therapist are what inspired me to write this book. The stories my patients have so bravely shared with me have led me to want more, to be better, and to make a change. Without my patients, there would be no book.

INTRODUCTION: WHY THIS BOOK

*"There is no force equal to
a woman determined to rise."*

—W.E.B. Dubois

It's about damn time we have a book dedicated to women for our needs between the hips! Welcome to this practical guide for women, which I've designed to inform you of what's really normal so you can finally get the help you deserve.

Have you been told that your discomfort "down there" is normal? Or that wetting your pants is just part of getting older, especially if you've experienced childbirth? Maybe you've even been told your symptoms are in your head. Well, guess what? They're not! It's NOT NORMAL to have pelvic discomfort, to leak (even just a drop), or to have any pelvic issues for that matter—babies or not.

This guide uses easy-to-follow descriptions and illustrations to walk you through the anatomy and physiology of everything between the hips. My goal is to help you understand what you weren't—but should have been!—taught as part of health classes, in anatomy and physiology classes, and during doctor appointments. The information in this book has the potential to change your life for the better. This guide will help you make sure that medical professionals understand your issues so you can get answers and find solutions. It will also encourage you to get the care and treatment you need and deserve.

Brace yourself. We have a lot to get through! Read this in order or skip around to the chapters most applicable to you. Whichever route you go, be sure to write down questions, comments, or concerns to discuss with your healthcare provider. The test-tracking log included in Appendix A can also help you stay organized. No question is a dumb question, and if you don't advocate for yourself, who will?

Before we continue, I do want to note that all physical therapists have their own style of treatment based on their experiences and interpretation of the medical and professional literature about symptoms and treatments. This book represents my style, experiences, and interpretation of the literature, and I acknowledge that other physical therapists may use different approaches that work for them. The bottom line, however, is that all physical therapists are working toward the same objective: helping patients achieve their goals.

Ladies, gals, women, superheroes: Enjoy the read and learn new information that can give you the quality of life you deserve!

YOU ARE NOT ALONE

As a Doctor of Physical Therapy specializing in pelvic health, I committed to becoming a Board-Certified Women's Health Clinical Specialist (WCS). My nearly yearlong study and preparation for this specialty certification was invaluable, and as a woman, I couldn't believe how unaware I had been of some of the essential information I was finally learning. Honestly, I was also angry. I was angry that prior to this time, I had not been able to obtain this information in an accessible, comprehensive way; angry that when I was a teenager, my doctor didn't explain to me the potential lifelong damage of eating disorders; angry that my emergency room visits for abdominal pain were chalked up to constipation and I was told simply to take a laxative; and angry that my doctor never asked at my yearly physicals if intercourse was painful.

I was especially saddened to discover that so many women are not being taken seriously and receiving the help they need. My patients—brave and courageous—have shared their stories with me, summarizing sometimes years of physical pain and emotional distress, being passed from one healthcare provider to another without answers and without being closer to a solution. I have cried and empathized with these women, and then as a result of their physical therapy treatment program, I have celebrated with them as they returned to living their life without pain and without pelvic floor dysfunction.

After becoming a Women's Health Clinical Specialist through the American Physical Therapy Association, I thought, "What am I going to do about it now?" This book, *Between the Hips,* is my answer. I hope this opens a platform for you and other women to know that YOU ARE NOT ALONE. Go tell your friends, shout it at the top of your lungs, and know there is help!

Society has shamed us as women into keeping quiet about issues between our hips, but not anymore. Now, through the knowledge of what is normal and what is not, you will have the power. It's about damn time, so let's begin!

CHAPTER ONE

The Pelvic Girdle

"The female pelvis is a powerhouse
of energy transformation, the very throne
of creation through which universal
creative energy patterns course and flow."

—Dr. Rosita Arvigo, DN

BEFORE I WOW YOU with the cool scientific details of the pelvic girdle, which sits between your hips, I need to explain why I am including this thick anatomy lesson up front. My aim here is to get across the point that there is a lot going on in your pelvic region. Consequently, if you are having pain or issues, ladies, please be patient with yourself and be kind to yourself! By no means do you need to memorize the material in this chapter. (It took me months to even learn how to pronounce and spell these muscles, let alone understand what they all do.) However, with that in mind, knowledge is power, so let's start by reviewing some of the basics here.

THE GIRDLE

The pelvis, also known as the pelvic girdle (similar in name and function to the undergarment worn by generations of women to hold their midsections tight), acts to hold everything between our hips together. Our pelvis is made up of a bony ring that includes the sacroiliac joints in the back and the pubic symphysis joint in the front. The pelvis connects to our spine above and to our hips at the sides, providing stability for everything we do. (See figure 1.) As girls go through puberty, their hips widen to eventually accommodate childbirth, thus women have a wider pelvis than men.

Figure 1: The Pelvic Girdle

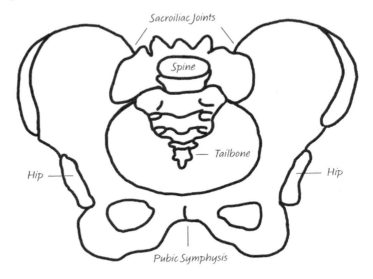

Sacroiliac Joints

Spine

Tailbone

Hip

Hip

Pubic Symphysis

Attached under the pelvic girdle is the pelvic floor, a group of muscles consisting of three layers that provide support to the internal organs. Above the pelvic girdle and under the rib cage sits the diaphragm. Between the diaphragm and pelvic girdle sit our core muscles. (They *are* there; I promise you that everyone has them!) Think of this area like a canister throughout the trunk of your body; in the canister everything is intertwined and connected.

Before we move on, let's talk briefly about the core. You may be surprised—and perhaps relieved—to know that even if you cannot see your core muscles it really doesn't matter, because the highly sought after "six-pack" muscle, which is called the rectus abdominis, really isn't the muscle you need to be the strongest. In the front, your core is made up of the oblique muscles that run diagonal along your rib cage; the rectus abdominis muscle, which spans from your breastbone to your pubic bone; and the transverse abdominis muscle, which wraps around your entire trunk like a corset, spanning to join the pelvic floor muscles behind your pubic bone. These muscles are illustrated in figure 2.

(Note: the oblique muscles are shown only on one side so the deeper transverse abdominis muscles can be viewed on the other side.) In the back, in addition to the transverse abdominis, your core is made up of spine stabilizer muscles. The transverse abdominis muscle is the key muscle to focus on because it is the deepest of the core muscles and it provides the pelvis and spine the most stability when working directly with the pelvic floor. Think of the pelvic floor muscles and the transverse abdominis muscle as best-friend muscles that help and support each other with everything. As you read this book, you will see just how codependent these two friendly muscles are.

Figure 2: The Core Muscles

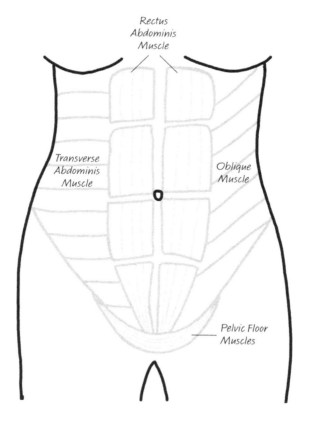

Rectus
Abdominis
Muscle

Transverse
Abdominis
Muscle

Oblique
Muscle

Pelvic Floor
Muscles

THE PELVIC FLOOR

The pelvic floor consists of three layers of muscles, which include thirteen muscles altogether. Most women have no idea of the vast role of these muscles and the effect they have on our daily life, so let's take a quick look.

Function

The pelvic floor serves four main functions:

1. *Support and stability.* These muscles support and stabilize our abdominal organs, bladder, uterus, ovaries, and rectum.
2. *Leakage prevention.* The sphincters close off the urethral and rectal openings to avoid accidental leaking of urine, stool, or gas.
3. *Sump pump action.* The muscles aid in the circulation of oxygen and nutrient-rich blood to help maintain healthy tissue. When they contract, especially during a Kegel exercise or during an orgasm, oxygen and nutrient-depleted blood is pushed out of the tissue while oxygen and nutrient-rich blood is drawn in. Because of the relationship between the hips and the pelvic floor, this exchange is also achieved through walking, stair climbing, or any other use of your legs.
4. *Sexual stimulation.* The muscles expand to accommodate vaginal penetration and they contract to aid in clitoral erection.

Muscle Fiber Types

Like all other muscles, the pelvic floor muscles are made up of Type 1 and Type 2 fibers. It is easiest to think of Type 1 and Type 2 muscle fibers in terms of running. Type 1 muscle fibers are responsible for sustained endurance, like a marathon; Type 2 muscle fibers are responsible for quick, short bursts, like a sprint. Understanding the characteristics of both fiber types will help you better train your pelvic floor, which we will discuss later in the "Weak Pelvic Floor Muscle" section of chapter 7, "To Lengthen or Strengthen." Table 1 distinguishes between the two fiber types.

Table 1: Muscle Fiber Types

TYPE 1 FIBERS	TYPE 2 FIBERS
• Slow-twitch 'marathon' fibers • Constant support to internal organs • Makes up 70 percent of the muscle fibers	• Fast-twitch 'sprint' fibers • Quick engagement for stability and continence • Makes up 30 percent of the muscle fibers

If you think about it, it makes perfect sense that our pelvic floor muscles have more Type 1 "marathon" fibers since the pelvic floor muscles must provide constant support throughout the day.

The Muscles

As mentioned earlier, there are three layers of pelvic floor muscles. The first and second layers of muscles are different vaginally versus rectally, while the third layer of muscles are the same vaginally and rectally. Don't feel overwhelmed here. After you take a look at Table 2, just remember one simple fact: there are a lot of muscles around your vagina.

Table 2: The Pelvic Floor Muscles

LAYER	MUSCLES	ROLE
First layer vaginally	Superficial transverse perineal Bulbocavernosus Ischiocavernosus	Promotes clitoral erection Assists with sphincter function of second layer
First layer rectally	External anal sphincter (EAS)	Contracts to maintain continence of stool and gas Relaxes to allow passage of stool and gas

(continued on next page)

(continued from previous page)

LAYER	MUSCLES	ROLE
Second layer vaginally	Deep transverse perineal Compressor urethrae Sphincter urethrovaginalis External urethral sphincter	Contracts to maintain continence of urine Relaxes to allow passage of urine
Second layer rectally	Internal anal sphincter (IAS)	Relaxes to provide "sample" of rectal contents to the external anal sphincter (see page 64 of chapter 5, "Bowel Health")
Third layer vaginally and rectally	Pubococcygeus: made from puborectalis and pubovaginalis Iliococcygeus Obturator internus Coccygeus The third layer is also known as the levator ani group	All: Provide support to the internal organs and stabilize the pelvic girdle with arm and leg movements Pubococcygeus: Contracts to elevate and close the anal canal; relaxes to allow stool to pass Obturator internus: Assists with hip rotation Coccygeus: Stabilizes the tailbone and sacrum

To put it all together, let's look at these muscles! Check out figure 3 to view the first layer of muscles, figure 4 to view the second layer of muscles, and figure 5 to view the third layer of muscles.

Figure 3: Pelvic Floor Muscles, Layer 1

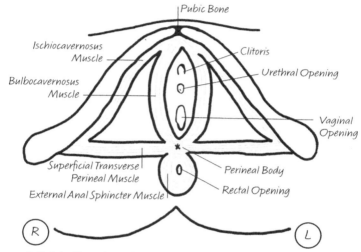

Figure 4: Pelvic Floor Muscles, Layer 2

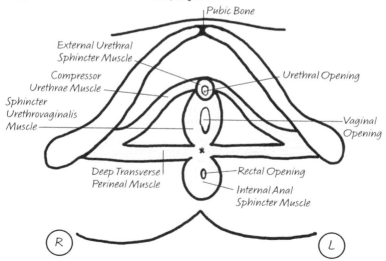

Figure 5: Pelvic Floor Muscles, Layer 3

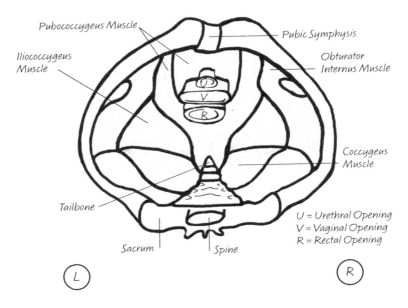

Pubococcygeus Muscle

Iliococcygeus Muscle

Pubic Symphysis

Obturator Internus Muscle

Coccygeus Muscle

Tailbone

U = Urethral Opening
V = Vaginal Opening
R = Rectal Opening

Sacrum

Spine

L

R

The Perineum

The perineum is not a specific muscle; instead, this term describes the outermost area of the genitals. The perineal body is a dense fibrous tissue that provides a central attachment point for the superficial pelvic floor muscles. It is located between the vaginal and rectal opening. The perineal body will be more elevated in a woman who has never given birth than in a woman who has given birth.

The perineal body is also a central dividing point for the front half of the pelvic floor (the urogenital triangle) and the back half of the pelvic floor (the anorectal triangle). As figure 6 shows, the urogenital triangle includes the vaginal and urethral opening, while the anorectal triangle includes the rectal opening. Within the urogenital triangle of the perineum is the vulva, which is the term for the tissue surrounding the vaginal opening. As you may know, the vagina is enclosed in two lip-like folds. The outermost fold is called the labia majora and the inner fold is called the labia minora. The labia begin at the pubic bone and span to the perineal body, encompassing and protecting the clitoris, urethral opening, and vaginal opening. This is also displayed in figure 6.

Figure 6: The Perineum Structures

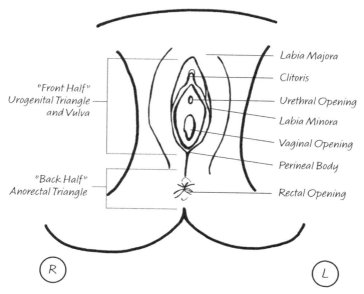

"Front Half"
Urogenital Triangle
and Vulva

"Back Half"
Anorectal Triangle

Labia Majora
Clitoris
Urethral Opening
Labia Minora
Vaginal Opening
Perineal Body
Rectal Opening

R   L

I am going to take a minute to promote a bit of self-love here. I encourage you to look up "The Great Wall of Vagina."[1] Here you will see that an artist made plaster casts of 400 women's vulvas and displayed them as a work of art. What you'll notice is that every single vulva looks different: whether the labia minora extend beyond the labia majora, the labia majora completely enclose the vulva, or the majora rest in a more open position——it is all okay! There is no standard as to what the vulva should look like, and, thus, there is no such thing as an ugly vagina. I've had a handful of women apologize to me during physical therapy sessions for having to view their "ugly" or "unflattering" vaginas. It breaks my heart to think some women are embarrassed or ashamed of how they look "down there," and I quickly educated them on this very topic. Remember, there is no standard, normal look we should desire to have.

Nerve Supply

Just like muscles anywhere else in the body, the pelvic floor muscles function from neural innervation, which is a fancy phrase for nerve supply. In other words, a nerve supplies the muscles with the ability to contract, relax, and sense. The pelvic floor muscles are supplied by two nerves. The first, the pudendal nerve, primarily supplies the first two muscle layers, while the second, the levator ani nerve, primarily supplies the third layer.

The pudendal nerve takes a complicated path from the back of the pelvis, weaving in and out and in again, eventually reaching the muscles. You might say it takes the long way home. The pudendal nerve starts from the back of your pelvis at the sacrum (see figure 7). The nerve spans from sacral level 2 (S2) through sacral level 4 (S4). In my world of physical therapy, this applies when we tell patients, "S2, S3, S4 keep pee and poop off the floor." The pudendal nerve then divides into three branches: the inferior rectal, middle perineal, and dorsal clitoral branch, as illustrated in figure 8. You might be wondering, "Why all the details on this nerve?" It goes back to the point that there is a lot that goes on in the pelvic region, and I want to give you an understanding of this nerve because we will be further discussing it on page 90 of chapter 6, "Pelvic Pain."

Figure 7: Pudendal Nerve at the Sacrum

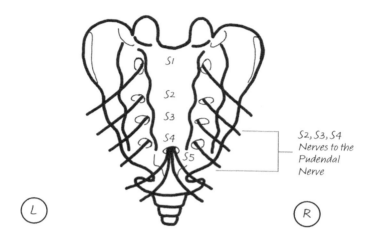

S1
S2
S3
S4
S5

S2, S3, S4
Nerves to the
Pudendal
Nerve

L

R

Figure 8: Pudendal Nerve Branches

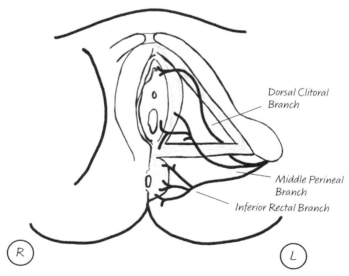

Dorsal Clitoral
Branch

Middle Perineal
Branch

Inferior Rectal Branch

R

L

The levator ani nerve also starts from the sacrum. Unlike the pudendal nerve, this nerve does not take a complicated path but instead heads straight for the levator ani muscle group, which is also referred to as the third layer of the pelvic floor muscles. See figure 9.

Figure 9: Levator Ani Nerve Branch

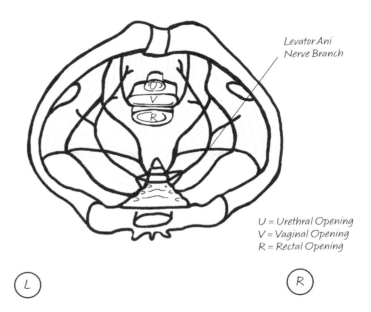

Levator Ani
Nerve Branch

U = Urethral Opening
V = Vaginal Opening
R = Rectal Opening

L   R

Glands

Think of the vestibule of a building: it is an area between the outside and inside of the building, like an entrance hall. Similarly, the vestibule of the pelvic floor is the entrance to the vaginal opening; it is the area just prior to the vaginal opening inside the labia minor (the inner lips). There are two types of vestibular glands associated with this area.

The greater vestibular glands (the Bartholin's glands) are located next to the vaginal opening and are responsible for secreting mucus to lubricate the vagina, especially during sexual arousal. The lesser vestibular glands (the Skene's glands) are located on the front portion of the vaginal wall by the urethra. Skene's glands assist with lubrication and blood flow during sexual arousal, and they are also thought to assist in protecting the urethral opening.

THE PELVIC ORGANS

The bladder, uterus, and rectum make up the pelvic organs, which are nuzzled into their respective spots, assisting and supporting each other as shown in figure 10.

When properly supported and positioned, the pelvic organs can function optimally. However, when the essential support system of the pelvic floor fails, dysfunction and pain frequently result. Let's continue to chapter 2, "When Your Pelvic Support System Fails," to learn more about this issue and ways to address it.

Figure 10: A Side View of the Pelvic Organs

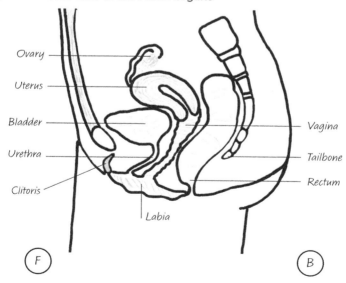

CHAPTER TWO

When Your Pelvic Support System Fails

*"When women support each other,
incredible things happen."*

—Unknown

Y OU MAY BE AWARE that a woman's bladder, urethra, uterus, and/or rectum can begin falling out of her vagina (this is referred to as a prolapse). But did you also know there are things you can do to decrease your risk of having this happen in the first place? There are even ways to help correct it if it already has happened. Better yet, did you know that just because you have a prolapse doesn't necessarily mean you need surgery? Sometimes, women who have a prolapse feel completely normal and have no issues! Let's delve in.

PELVIC ORGAN PROLAPSE (POP)

The pelvic floor muscles and other tissues, along with healthy nerve supply, assist to support the pelvic organs. As mentioned above, pelvic organ prolapse (POP) occurs when the bladder, urethra, uterus, and/or rectum lacks support and begins falling out of the vagina. Here are more details.

Symptoms of POP

Common symptoms of POP include the following:

1. You feel a bulge, pelvic pressure, or pelvic heaviness that is more prominent with straining.
2. You experience aching in your lower back because ligaments and fascia are straining to support the prolapsed, falling organ.

15

3. You notice bleeding, discharge, or infections as a result of increased friction of the prolapse.
4. You feel better in the morning versus in the evening. As the day goes on, gravity further causes the organ to fall and prolapse more out of the vagina.
5. During intercourse, you experience pelvic or abdominal pain because the prolapsed organ can block vaginal penetration. When the prolapsed organ is bumped, it can be painful.

If your bladder is prolapsed, you might experience a poor or prolonged urine stream, a feeling of incomplete bladder emptying, a need to change positions to start or complete emptying, and dribbling leaks after voiding. In contrast, if your rectum is prolapsed (as shown in figure 11), you might experience feeling like you haven't emptied your bowels completely, and you may be forced to use splinting, a technique some women use to fully empty their bowels by using their thumb inserted vaginally to push backward toward the tailbone. Figure 12 shows exactly how splinting works. If you experience symptoms of POP and struggle with complete bowel emptying, you may wish to try this splinting technique at the end of your bowel movement. A pelvic floor physical therapist can provide further education to help you know if this is an appropriate action for you, and if it is, offer instructions to do so.

CAUSES OF PELVIC ORGAN PROLAPSE

You might be wondering what contributes to developing POP in the first place. Common factors include the following:

1. *The Valsalva maneuver:* Holding your breath during physical exertion such as pushing, pulling, or lifting is referred to as the Valsalva maneuver. When you hold your breath during exertion, no air escapes through your nose or mouth, which places excess force through your abdomen. In contrast, when you exhale through your nose or mouth during physical exertion, less stress is placed through your abdomen, which is kinder and gentler for your pelvic organs.

Figure 11: Rectal Prolapse

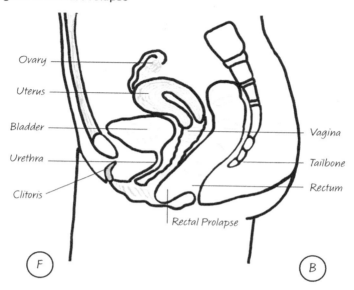

Ovary

Uterus

Bladder

Urethra

Clitoris

Vagina

Tailbone

Rectum

Rectal Prolapse

F

B

Figure 12: Splinting for Rectal Prolapse

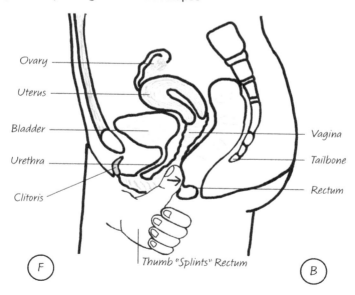

Ovary

Uterus

Bladder

Urethra

Clitoris

Vagina

Tailbone

Rectum

Thumb "Splints" Rectum

F

B

2. *Constipation:* With excessive straining and pushing, especially if you are using the Valsalva maneuver described previously, you place increased stress on the abdominal cavity. (Refer to page 70 for ways to address constipation.)

3. *Pregnancy:* Pregnancy places increased demands on the pelvic floor to support the weight of the growing baby. With vaginal deliveries, the risk of POP increases when there is excessive straining to push using a Valsalva technique, perineal tearing, and/or deliveries assisted with vacuums or forceps. For more information, check out chapter 8, "Pregnancy."

4. *Chronic coughing:* Excessive coughing with a bad cold, smoking, or chronic obstructive pulmonary disease places excessive demand on the pelvic floor to support the organs against an increase in abdominal pressure. This is especially true if you are not doing the knack while coughing. Doing the knack involves squeezing to engage your pelvic floor muscles and core muscles prior to coughing. This provides support to your internal organs by lifting your bladder and closing the urethra to brace against the abdominal force of the cough. The knack is a key technique! We'll talk a lot more about the knack on page 51 of chapter 4, "Bladder Health," and on page 111 of chapter 7, "To Lengthen or Strengthen."

5. *Obesity:* Carrying extra weight increases stress and demand on the pelvic floor for support. Current thinking suggests that losing 5 to 10 percent of your body weight can help decrease POP symptoms.[2]

6. *Poor posture:* Slouching increases the pressure on the pelvic organs, and it decreases the support from the muscles. Sit up straight, ladies!

7. *Collagen defects:* Tissue laxity, as seen with tissue disorders like Benign Joint Hypermobility Syndrome (BJHS) and Ehlers-Danlos Syndrome, leads to decreased support of the pelvic organs.

8. *Estrogen deficiency:* During menopause, a decrease in estrogen production causes thinning of tissues. This leads to decreased strength

and support of connective tissue for the pelvic organs. (Refer to page 156 of chapter 10, "Life Stages and Pelvic Health," for more information on menopausal changes.)

9. *Hysterectomy:* Removing the uterus contributes to POP because the bladder and rectum lose the support of the uterus and fill in the space left by the uterus. Unfortunately, your body does not hold a memorial site for the uterus. (See figure 13.) Without adequate pelvic floor support, the bladder and/or rectum can begin falling into the vagina.

Figure 13: Lack of Support with a Hysterectomy

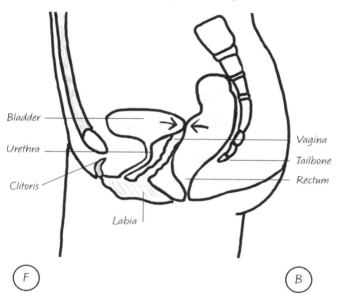

TYPES OF PELVIC ORGAN PROLAPSE

There are many combinations of prolapses that can occur. Table 3 provides names and descriptions.

Table 3: Types of Pelvic Organ Prolapse

PROLAPSE NAME	DESCRIPTION
Cystocele	Bladder is falling into the front of the vaginal wall.
Urethrocele	Urethra is falling into the front of the vaginal wall.
Urethrocystocele	Bladder and urethra are falling into the front of the vaginal wall.
Rectocele	Rectum is falling into the back of the vaginal wall.
Enterocele	Small intestines are falling into the back of the vaginal wall.
Vaginal Vault	Top of the vagina is falling down on itself.
Uterine	Uterus is falling down along the vaginal wall.
Rectal	Rectum is falling down on itself.

As mentioned previously, even if you do have a prolapse, you may be completely symptom free. In that case, you should take specific actions to avoid making the prolapse worse; otherwise, you may start experiencing symptoms. For example, if you are symptom free, then as a precaution you should avoid the Valsalva maneuver and take steps to prevent constipation. Regardless of the type of prolapse or degree of symptoms you may be experiencing, a pelvic floor physical therapist can help guide you in the right direction. Let's take a look at some specific treatment options next.

TREATMENT FOR PELVIC ORGAN PROLAPSE

The treatment options that are available depend on the severity of the prolapse. As the following list shows, pelvic organ prolapse can vary in severity from Grade 1 to Grade 4:

Grade 1: The distended organ is halfway down the vaginal opening.

Grade 2: The distended organ is at the vaginal opening.

Grade 3: The distended organ is halfway below the vaginal opening.

Grade 4: The distended organ is completely outside the vaginal opening.

Usually with a Grade 4 POP, you will require surgery. However, while the surgery will correct the pelvic organ prolapse, it will not correct the habits and behaviors that contributed to it, so physical therapy is still warranted and necessary! In fact, by addressing the habits and behaviors that led to the prolapse in the first place, pelvic floor physical therapy can help ensure that the surgery is successful and help prevent reoccurrence.

For less severe cases, pelvic floor physical therapy alone, without surgery, has been shown to help reverse milder grades of prolapse.[3] Let's look at how that can happen.

The first step is to get a referral to a physical therapist who specializes in pelvic floor treatment. (Again, this should be done whether or not you need or have had surgery.) First, your therapist will get to know you and your symptoms. Then, if you are comfortable with it, they will perform a one-gloved-finger vaginal and/or rectal pelvic floor muscle assessment. If your muscles present as tight and painful, then the goal of the physical therapy is to first relax and lengthen the muscles. As appropriate, the therapist will work with you on strengthening the muscles. Ultimately, by first relaxing (if needed) and then strengthening your pelvic floor muscles, you'll find that pelvic floor physical therapy will result in better support for your pelvic organs, which should relieve your discomfort and pain. To put it more bluntly: Kegels are not the one-stop-shop solution!

Sometimes, other treatment needs to be done first. Check out chapter 7, "To Lengthen or Strengthen," to learn even more!

When you are ready, your physical therapist will provide you with several ways to strengthen your pelvic floor muscles. The treatment may include a combination of the following:

- *Explaining the benefits of and the correct ways to do Kegel exercises.* Kegel exercises involve squeezing to engage only your core and pelvic floor muscles to specifically isolate and strengthen your pelvic floor. Doing a correct Kegel can be tricky because there are several ways your body will want to cheat. For example, squeezing your inner-thigh muscles and your butt-cheek muscles are common ways to cheat. When you do that, you are no longer isolating just the pelvic floor muscles but rather pulling in other muscles to help.
- *Demonstrating the use of vaginal weights, if indicated.* Small vaginal weights can be used to further strengthen your pelvic floor. This approach is similar to how holding a weight in your hand can further strengthen your arm muscles. However, because it is easy to cheat and use other muscles besides your pelvic floor to hold the weight in, vaginal weights aren't for everyone.
- *Giving you hip-strengthening exercises.* These are beneficial because the hips and pelvic floor are so closely related. Remember, the obturator internus muscle of the third layer assists with hip rotation. Strengthening the hips can thus help strengthen the pelvic floor.

If your situation does not require surgery or you would like to try a conservative, nonsurgical option first, an elastic or rigid device called a *pessary* can assist in decreasing the symptoms of a prolapse. A pessary, which is individually fitted to you by your gynecologist, is inserted vaginally and acts to lift and support the prolapsed organ. If you are able to, you can remove the pessary yourself at home for cleaning roughly every three months and then reinsert it. However, this timing varies, and your gynecologist will provide you with very specific guidelines to follow. You can leave a pessary in place during intercourse, but some women and partners find them uncomfortable. If that is your experience, then it is important to learn how to remove and reinsert it on your own at home. If you are unable to remove and reinsert it yourself, then you will need to schedule appointments with your gynecologist for this.

Pessaries come in many shapes and sizes, as seen in figure 14. Although using a pessary does not fix the prolapse, it can help you with managing your symptoms. Your gynecologist can assist you in a pessary fitting and management.

Figure 14: Types of Pessaries

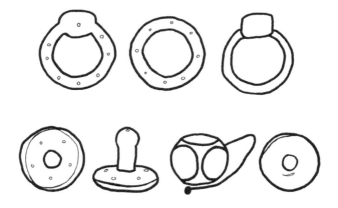

Lifestyle modification is an absolute must for prolapse management whether or not you require surgery. As noted earlier, some of the contributing factors to prolapse include coughing, constipation, the Valsalva maneuver, and obesity. You must address these behaviors in order to decrease the risk of worsening your symptoms. Even if you require surgery to correct your prolapse and it is fixed, the prolapse can return if you continue to excessively strain with bowel movements or use the Valsalva maneuver with lifting. It is important to identify why the prolapse happened in the first place and take action to correct these behaviors. A pelvic floor physical therapist will help you with the necessary lifestyle modifications so you can start to get your pelvic health back on track.

CHAPTER THREE

Between the Hips Sexy Self-Care

"Self-care is the best care."

—Unknown

NERVOUS ABOUT ODORS DOWN THERE? Do you want to learn what actually happens during an orgasm and what type of lubricant is best for you? Are you curious to learn about the best way to pee in a public bathroom? Did you know that painful periods are not normal? Welcome to chapter 3!

HYGIENE

The vagina is like a self-cleaning oven that you don't even need to start or program. Let it clean itself! The genital area is made of delicate, sensitive tissue. Washing this area with soaps, fragrances, or detergents can throw off the pH balance and the natural vaginal flora while also contributing to pain, itching, and irritation. To clean this area, separate the labia minor (the inner lips) and bathe the tissue with lukewarm water using only your hand; do not wash into the vagina, just the inner lip area. When done, let the lips fold together and gently pat the outer lips dry with a towel. This area should not be washed more than once a day to decrease irritation, although it is not even necessary to wash it daily.

I know what you might be thinking: you're worried about "smelling bad down there." It is normal and natural for the genitals to have a slight odor, so trying to rid yourself of this natural fragrance may be doing more harm than good. However, if you have a foul, fishy odor, do consult your doctor to test for infections.

If you find you are experiencing genital irritation, here are some things to try:

- Wear white cotton underwear.
- Use soft, white unscented toilet paper.
- Switch to fragrance-free laundry detergent.
- Use organic, unscented, and unbleached tampons and pads or try menstrual cups, which are discussed later in this chapter.

Be mindful that swimsuits, hot tubs, cycling, tight-fitting clothing, lubricants, saliva, condoms, and bowel and bladder leakage can also irritate the genital area.

TAKING A LOOK

Have you ever actually held a mirror and looked "down there"? I'm going to guess that most of you haven't, likely because you've never been educated as to why you should or because you may be bashful. Let's change this—and here's why!

As you become familiar with what your perineum, vulva, labia, vaginal opening, and rectal opening all look like, you can catch any potential issue sooner and monitor changes over time. Look to see if the tissue appears to be red, irritated, or dry. Check for hemorrhoids (which we will discuss on page 83 of chapter 5, "Bowel Health") and POPs, which appear as a bulge descending from your vagina. You may also notice that your urethral opening is becoming pale in color, which can occur during menopause (discussed on page 157), or that your labia are becoming darker in color, which can occur with pelvic pain (discussed on page 96).

You can complete this self-examination standing up or lying down, whichever is most comfortable for you. If you are standing, place one foot up on a closed toilet lid; if you are lying on a bed, spread your legs with your knees bent and place your feet flat on the bed. With one hand, hold a small mirror between your thighs and use your other hand to investigate. Be sure you spread your labia so you can thoroughly view all of the tissue: clitoris, urethral opening, and vaginal opening. Lastly, spread your butt cheeks in the back so you can view your rectal opening. Just like you wipe from front to back, you'll view from front to back. Pick a time once a month to do this and try to make it a day you'll remember, such as the first day of the month or the day you do your monthly breast exam (which is discussed on page 165 of the bonus chapter at the end of this book).

THE DREADED PUBLIC RESTROOM

Here's a quick rhyme you can refer to whenever you need to use a public restroom: *nest is best; squat is not!* Up to this point in time, you may have been thinking, "If I'm peeing in a public bathroom, it's okay to squat, right? I mean, who wants to actually sit down, exposing your bare bum to so many gross bathroom germs?" Well, actually, squatting is not acceptable, and it's not good for your bladder or your pelvic floor muscles. Let me tell you why!

When you squat, your pelvic floor muscles are tense, so they cannot relax. This makes it harder for your bladder to initiate the urine flow, which means you may have to push a bit to start the stream. That's also when the trouble starts. Pushing can lead to pelvic organ prolapse, which we've discussed earlier. Additionally, because you are tensing your muscles, squatting can confuse the neurological reflex that traditionally starts the flow of urine only when your muscles relax.

As much as I love a good leg workout, don't do your squats in the bathroom. Put clean toilet paper down on the seat to make a more hygienic nest. Then sit, relax, and let your body do its job.

ORGASMS

We absolutely have to talk about orgasms. Can you ever recall being taught what happens during a female orgasm or how an orgasm is achieved? Probably not. Why is there so little information on this topic for women? This imbalance likely stems from gender stereotyping, where societal stigmas have made women feel as if they cannot ask for or express what they want.[4] According to research, during intercourse 95 percent of men achieve an orgasm while just 65 percent of women achieve an orgasm,[5] and up to 50 percent of women fake achieving an orgasm.[6]

Just because a woman does not experience an orgasm, this does not mean she cannot experience sexual pleasure. However, if this is a challenge for you, understanding the science behind an orgasm may help you better achieve an orgasm in addition to sexual pleasure.

An orgasm occurs when there is a surge in blood flow to the genital area along with spontaneous pelvic floor muscle contractions that occur faster and faster and faster until climax (orgasm). Remember, as we discussed in chapter 1, one role of the pelvic floor muscles is to act as a "sump pump" to aid in bringing oxygen-rich blood and nutrient-rich blood to the pelvis to help keep tissues healthy. When a woman achieves an orgasm, the sump pump function is successful, and new oxygen-rich blood and nutrient-rich blood are delivered to the pelvis.

Orgasm can be achieved by vaginal penetration, clitoral stimulation, vaginal and clitoral stimulation, breast stimulation, or erotic thoughts. However, research indicates that most women require some degree of clitoral stimulation to orgasm.[7] The clitoris has 8,000 nerve endings and is much larger than the eye can see, extending internally past the vaginal opening. (See figure 15.) Because we all are different, it makes sense that an orgasm can be achieved and expressed differently by everyone.

Believe it or not, women can experience several orgasms (contrary to men, who experience only one). In fact, once you achieve your first orgasm, you may be able to more easily achieve another and another. This is because after you've achieved your first orgasm, the female genitals continue to be hyper-responsive and sensitive to stimulation. Thus, you may experience multiple, more intense orgasms.[8]

But wait, what about "The G-spot"? What does that even stand for or mean beyond a term referenced in dirty rap songs? The G-spot is thought to be a spot on the front wall of the vagina that, when stimulated, can result in an orgasm. It gets its name from the doctor who is credited with discovering it, Dr. Gräfenberg. As stated previously, to achieve orgasm you may require clitoral stimulation and vaginal stimulation, thought to be at the G-spot. However, it is up for debate whether or not the G-spot even exists.[9] You can be the judge!

Figure 15: Clitoral Anatomy

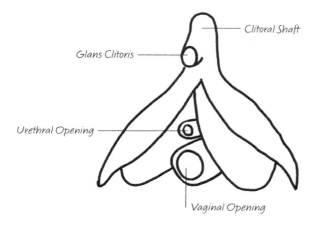

Okay, ladies, now that you understand the basic science behind orgasms, some of you may be thinking, "Shoot, I don't have a partner to help me achieve this." Hello! That's what masturbation is for. Masturbation can help improve intensity and frequency of orgasms because it allows you to discover what feels the best. (And if you do have a partner, you can use your findings to better communicate what feels good and what you need to do to achieve orgasm.) Some people view masturbation as a negative act, a sin, or evil. I strongly disagree. There should be no shame in self-pleasure, and it even does your pelvic floor good. Why should women have to rely on someone else for sexual fulfillment? My best bit of advice for you is to experiment, communicate, and shamelessly love yourself for whatever route is needed to achieve your best orgasm. I highly recommend you watch the documentary *Explained: The Female Orgasm* to learn more about orgasm![10]

Of note, there are several factors that can contribute to lack of orgasms. Some examples include pelvic pain, history of trauma, emotional factors, and environmental and situational circumstances. Check out chapter 6, "Pelvic Pain," for further discussion on specifics to pelvic pain. You may also find it beneficial to consult a behavioral therapist or sex therapist to further delve into your unique needs to help you achieve orgasm and pleasurable intercourse.

LUBRICANTS

I recommend that everyone use lubricant liberally. It can help make your sexual experience much more pleasurable. But just what kind should you use? There are three main types of lubricants, so let's take a look at the pros and cons of each category:

Water-based (e.g., Astroglide and K-Y Jelly): These lubricants may or may not contain glycerin, which has a sweet taste to it. With glycerin, there is an increased risk for vaginal infections and irritation. Water-based lubricants are safe to use with condoms and will not stain fabric. However, they do dry up and become sticky over time. Check out the Good Clean Love brand for certified safe and organic water-based lubricants.[11]

Oil-based (e.g., coconut oil, avocado oil, or olive oil) or synthetic oil-based (e.g., mineral oils or Vaseline): You may conveniently have several of these oil-based lubricants in your home already. However, these lubricants may irritate your skin and stain fabric; they will also break down condoms. If you do choose to use an oil-based lubricant, then coconut oil, avocado oil, or olive oil is recommended over synthetic options.

Silicone-based (e.g., Replens or Überlube): Silicone-based lubricants are hypoallergenic, are safe to use with condoms, are the best lubricant to use in the shower, and last the longest, requiring less reapplication. However because they break down silicone, they are not recommended for use with silicone sex toys or silicone pelvic floor muscle stretching tools.

Overall, when you are choosing a lubricant, avoid fragrances and warming components, both of which can be irritating to the vaginal tissue. Also, use an ample amount to ensure maximum comfort.

CONTRACEPTIVES AND MENSTRUAL CUPS

I highly recommend that all women should read the book *Taking Charge of Your Fertility* by Toni Weschler.[12] She will help you understand everything there is to know about your menstrual cycle and your fertility signs, which will help you both when you are trying to conceive and when you are trying to avoid conceiving. I have learned more from her book on this topic than I have in any other text or class. When managed well by your provider, many contraceptives can suit your needs perfectly. However, although discussion on specific contraceptives is outside the scope of this book, it is important to know that certain methods of contraception can contribute to pelvic pain. Intrauterine devices (IUDs) can irritate the uterine lining, and hormonal birth controls (e.g., pills or implants) can increase the risk for vaginal infections. I know this because I've experienced these issues firsthand but was not warned or educated on these side effects by the provider. If you experience pelvic pain, please refer to chapter 6.

In the rest of this section, I want to share my thoughts on menstrual products, specifically menstrual cups. Menstrual cups, which are reusable silicone cups that you insert vaginally to catch menstrual fluid, are an eco-friendly alternative to tampons and pads. They also offer a huge cost savings over traditional products, and they are better for the environment. Cups can be left in for up to twelve hours, day and night, which is convenient because if you time it right, you only need to change them at home versus at work or school.

When you insert the cup vaginally, it forms a seal around the vaginal wall to catch all contents. After removal, you dump the contents into the toilet, clean the cup with soap and water, rinse it well, let it air dry if you are no longer using it, or reuse it by inserting it vaginally (no need to dry if you're going to reuse it right away). Cups come in different sizes and styles, and using them does take some serious practice.

Despite these great benefits, there are a few precautions to mention to ensure you are fully informed. Specifically, let's take a closer look at the removal of the cup. As mentioned, the cup creates a seal around the vaginal wall. During removal, this seal must be broken, and if that is done incorrectly, it may contribute to pelvic organ prolapse.[13] As we learned, POP occurs when the bladder, urethra, uterus, and/or rectum begins falling out of the vagina. Essentially, if you remove the cup incorrectly by pulling on the cup *before* breaking the seal, then there is a downward pull from the suction on the pelvic organs. Instead, when removing the cup, you must release the suctioned seal *prior to pulling the cup out.* You can release the suctioned seal by squeezing the bottom of the cup so the rim of the cup folds to break the suctioned seal. You can also insert your finger to the rim of the cup to break the seal. I personally love the FLEX cup for the easy pull-tab that breaks the seal for removal.[14]

Another concern is pelvic pain. I do want to stress that if you have pelvic pain and find that tampons are painful or uncomfortable to use, then it's likely that cups will be painful for you too. This is because with pelvic pain, usually there is a degree of pelvic floor muscle tightness and irritability. When inserting a cup or tampon vaginally, the pelvic floor muscles need to be able to stretch and relax around it, which can be painful. Please see chapter 6 for further discussion on this topic.

As you can see, there are pros and cons with use of a menstrual cup. Personally, I have found the initial adjustment period of getting comfortable with the FLEX cup to be worth it in the long run. This will not be the case for everyone, and that is okay! Try different options, and use the information in this section to decide what is best for you: tampon, cup, or pad.

CHAPTER FOUR

Bladder Health

"Dancing is fun, except when it's the potty dance.
We must demonstrate mind over bladder."

—Dr. Megan Rorabeck, DPT, WCS

THE BLADDER IS A fascinating muscular organ, but it can develop bad habits and a mind of its own. Did you know that your bladder gives you signals as it fills and that it should signal you to pee every two to four hours? It can also be a bit quirky. For instance, have you ever experienced a sudden urge to pee right when you got home or when you heard the sound of running water, even though just a moment beforehand you felt no such urge? Maybe you even leak, especially after drinking a strong cup of joe or enjoying a cocktail. The bad news is that strong urges to pee, frequent peeing, and leaking (even just a tiny drop) are not normal bladder habits. The good news is that they can be changed! In fact, bladder habits can usually be changed by addressing your behaviors—not by doing Kegels. Keep reading to find out how.

ANATOMY

The bladder is a muscular organ designed to hold and store about two cups of urine. When your bladder fills, it relaxes, expanding and stretching to accommodate urine. When you pee, the bladder squeezes to empty, returning to its resting size. The inner lining of the bladder is a mucosal membrane like the lining of your mouth, and it can be sensitive to certain foods and fluids, which we will discuss shortly!

Once urine leaves your bladder, it has a three- to four-millimeter journey—only one eighth of an inch!—through the urethra to be emptied into the toilet. On each end of the urethra, you have a muscle. Closest to the bladder there is an internal sphincter muscle, and furthest from the bladder there is an external sphincter muscle. These sphincter muscles close off the urethra, working with the pelvic floor muscles to avoid leaking (see figure 16).

It is important to note that if you struggle with constipation, your bladder may be affected. With constipation, there is excess stool sitting in the rectum. This takes up space, leaving less room for your bladder to stretch to fill, store, and hold urine. If you experience bladder issues in conjunction with constipation, refer to the next chapter, "Bowel Health," to learn how to manage your constipation, which in turn will also help your bladder.

Figure 16: Female Bladder Anatomy

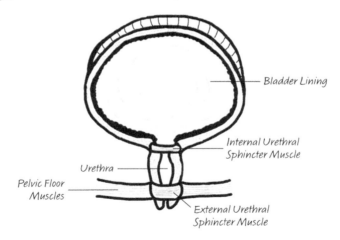

Bladder Lining

Internal Urethral Sphincter Muscle

Urethra

Pelvic Floor Muscles

External Urethral Sphincter Muscle

WHAT IS NORMAL

As noted, the bladder is designed to hold and store urine. In general, normal voiding occurs every two to four hours (five to seven times per day) and not at all or only one time at night. With that in mind, please note that certain medications, such as diuretics, can affect your bladder, which may contribute to strong urges, frequent voiding, bladder leakage, and other dysfunctions. If you find that this is the case, please consult directly with your physician for questions on this matter.

As a guideline, an easy and even fun way to check in with your bladder is to see if you pee for a stream of at least ten "Mississippis." If you make it to ten or beyond, then your bladder was truly full and thus it was appropriate for you to go. Yes, I did just say *appropriate to go,* because sometimes you will be tempted to pee when you shouldn't do so. Before you decide I am crazy, continue reading so I can explain.

HOW THE BLADDER WORKS

The bladder and pelvic floor muscles work together such that when you need to pee but aren't by a toilet, your pelvic floor muscles naturally squeeze, like when you're trying to hold back urine, and a message is sent to your bladder to relax. In contrast, when you sit on the toilet to pee, your pelvic floor muscles relax, and a message is sent to your bladder to squeeze and empty. This is called a reciprocal relationship; it is also called an opposite relationship, which is known as "Bradley's Loop." Bradley's Loop is a nervous system connection between your brain, spinal cord, bladder, and pelvic floor muscles. Figure 17, on the next page, illustrates just how this works.

Now, let's take a look at when it's appropriate to pee by exploring the signal program:

1. *The first signal:* When your bladder is filling, you get a first signal to pee when it's about one-third full. Your bladder is saying, "Hi, just so you know, I'm starting to fill." This should not cause an urgent need to stop what you're doing to pee; you can ignore this signal.

Figure 17: Reciprocal Relationship of the Pelvic Floor Muscles and Bladder

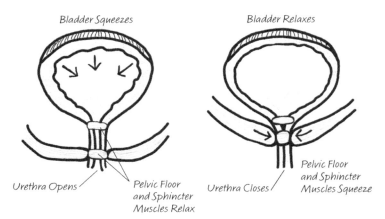

Bladder Squeezes

Bladder Relaxes

Urethra Opens

Pelvic Floor and Sphincter Muscles Relax

Urethra Closes

Pelvic Floor and Sphincter Muscles Squeeze

2. *The second signal:* Once your bladder fills a bit more, just over halfway or so, it will give you a second signal, saying, "You might want to start thinking about a plan to go." Again, this shouldn't cause an urgent need to pee, and maybe if you're super-focused on a project, you forget about the urge. Bottom line: start making a plan to go soon, and if this signal is strong, go now.

3. *The third signal:* If you ignore the second signal, this third signal will be stronger, and your bladder will likely be saying, "Time to go now!" This does not mean you should run to the toilet, as you will likely leak. (You will never outrun your bladder; trust me.) Stop what you're doing and calmly walk to the bathroom; unfasten your pants, shorts, or skirt in a controlled manner; sit down; and then start to pee.

Take a look at figure 18 to see how the bladder looks as it fills. It's also important to stay hydrated with good fluids, like water, so that you're getting appropriate signals. The "Bladder Irritants" section of this chapter discusses in greater detail how fluids affect your bladder.

Figure 18: The Bladder as It Fills

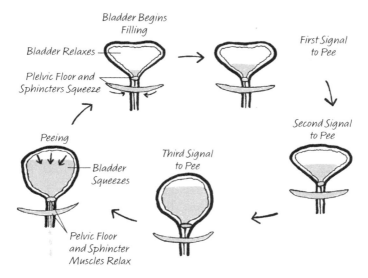

Our bladder has receptors so that the peeing process can work smoothly. If you always listen to the first signal and pee right away, then your bladder will lose its ability to stretch and hold urine, which can lead to problems such as leaking, experiencing strong urges, and frequently needing to pee. In addition, if you're peeing "just in case" or when you truly don't have to go (maybe out of convenience, such as that one last time before you get on the plane or into the car), you run the risk of resetting your bladder receptors, which occurs when your signal program gets thrown off. Instead of getting a normal third signal to go when your bladder is truly full, you will get a very strong signal when it's only partially full, causing you to pee at the first signal. This can all be very confusing to your bladder, but—good news—you can retrain it!

Now, I know what you might be thinking. It's never really that easy, right? I must be crazy for asking you to ignore the first two signals, to get to the bathroom calmly without running, and to avoid peeing "just in case." After all, didn't Mom always tell the kids to pee before sending them out to the car? Before you panic, though, let's talk about some common problems (and associated solutions) that occur during the peeing process.

Feeling Out of Control

Running, potty dancing, peeing before you've fully sat down, and leaking are all bad bladder habits. When you hustle and try running to the bathroom, you're more prone to leaking because you enter the "fight or flight" state of the sympathetic nervous system. As I've mentioned, you will never outrun your bladder. I've tried it and I know firsthand; I had pee all down my legs. I'm not trying to make light of the situation because it is incredibly embarrassing, but ladies, I've been there! Feeling out of control and leaking can happen to women of all ages. So, instead of running and panicking, *stay calm*. This will help you stay in the parasympathetic nervous system state of "rest and digest," where you will be better able to maintain control of your bladder.

Next time you get a sudden, strong urge to pee, try this process:

1. Stop and be still! Just for a few seconds, pause to calm your mind and your bladder. If you're standing, stand still; if you're sitting, stay sitting; if you're walking, stop. I know this sounds backward, but it is important to stop and calm your body to regain control. While stopping, talk yourself off the ledge of leaking. Try repeating these mantras:

   a. *I'm in control.*

   b. *Mind over bladder.*

   c. *Bladder, I didn't say it was time yet.*

   d. *I've got this. I'm almost at the toilet.*

   e. *Not now bladder.*

   There is value in positive self-talk, so give some love to yourself and your bladder. If you think negatively, such as saying to yourself, "Oh shoot, here I go again about to pee my pants," then guess what? You'll likely leak. Remain calm, stay positive, and be kind to yourself.

2. Once you've regained control, meaning the urge has calmed down a bit and you feel confident that you won't leak, *walk* calmly to the bathroom. If the urge sneaks up on you again along the way, repeat the process of stopping, being still, and regaining control. I literally mean that even if you're in the bathroom about to unfasten your pants and you're about to leak, then you must repeat the process: you must stop! If you rush and unfasten your pants but start to pee before you sit down, then you are just teaching your bladder that it's the one really in control.

Pushing to Pee

Pushing to pee is an approach you should avoid. If you push to pee, you risk causing a prolapse and your organs can start falling out of your vagina. (Please see the discussions about pelvic organ prolapse in chapter 2.) My patients usually tell me they push to pee because they are in a hurry to get back to what they're doing: taking care of the kids, cooking dinner, or working on a project for a client. Ladies, it can all wait! Remember Bradley's Loop, the reflex that sends a message to squeeze the bladder when the pelvic floor muscles relax? Well, this reflex is also responsible for helping your bladder squeeze long enough and hard enough to fully empty. To let the reflex do its job, you shouldn't push to pee. Bathroom time is *your* time: sit down, relax, and let your body do the work.

At times, you might feel the need to push to pee to start the flow of urine. This can be due to having tight pelvic floor muscles. Remember that the pelvic floor muscles need to relax to send the message to the bladder to squeeze to empty; this is the reciprocal relationship. If your pelvic floor muscles cannot relax as they should, then your bladder will have a hard time generating a strong enough squeeze to overcome the tension within the pelvic floor muscles, making you feel the need to push. So, just what can you do about this? When you sit on the toilet to pee, don't push. (It will be hard to break this habit.) Instead, try to relax, taking deep, calming breaths. Imagine your pelvic floor muscles—the area between your hips—softening, letting go, lengthening, or melting.

Use any analogy you want as long as it has a calming and relaxing effect to help get your muscles to relax so your bladder can then squeeze. (For more information on tight pelvic floor muscles, see chapter 7, "To Lengthen or Strengthen.")

Another reason you may need to push to pee can stem from waiting too long to pee. Now, this is not an excuse to be peeing every hour or just in case! I can hear some of you now: "Megan said I shouldn't wait too long to pee." No, I'm talking about waiting six-plus hours to pee. Believe it or not, I've seen it—with those in healthcare and education especially, because of their busy schedules and lack of time to go. So, they need to push to pee not only because their bladder is overstretched, but also because they're in a hurry to get back to their patients or students. I once treated a nurse who waited seventeen hours between peeing because she didn't have time to go! Being in healthcare myself, I get it. However, at the end of the day, *your* health is important too. How can you continue treating patients, teaching students, taking care of your children, crushing sales goals, or effectively doing whatever your job consists of if you don't take care of yourself? And dang it, good bathroom habits are important. Taking an extra minute in the bathroom won't hurt you or anyone else who relies on you.

Now that I've gotten that out, I can explain what actually happens when you wait too long to pee. As I've noted, the bladder stretches to fill and store and then squeezes to empty, returning to its resting size when it empties. Think of the bladder like a rubber band stretching to fill and then recoiling to empty. Now imagine if the rubber band is overstretched; it loses its elasticity and cannot recoil as easily. This is what can happen to the bladder if it is too full. It loses its ability to recoil and squeeze; thus, you may need to push to pee, using the force from your abdomen to help compress your bladder. As I've mentioned, usually you will get multiple signals to pee prior to this point, so be aware of your signals, and if you've hit the third signal, then go.

Feeling Incomplete Bladder Emptying

If you've ever noticed a dribble of pee on the toilet seat or feel like you have to pee again ten minutes after you just went, you might not be fully emptying your bladder. Incomplete emptying can stem from rushing yourself in the bathroom and pushing to pee; if you feel this is the case, then reread the previous section and remember that bathroom time is your time. Relax and take your time! If you're rushing, you may cut yourself off because you may decide that you've already sat on the toilet for too long and need to get back to what you're doing. This makes your bladder angry! Imagine if you're eating your favorite dessert and two bites in, someone snatches it away, saying, "You're done; get back to work." You'd be angry too. So again, give yourself the time you need and don't rush. In the long run, it will actually *save* you time because you won't have to go back to the bathroom ten minutes later to fully empty your bladder.

Incomplete emptying can also be due to a prolapse if your bladder and/or urethra is tilting into your vaginal canal. As figure 19 shows, this causes urine to get stuck in your bladder. Also see chapter 2, "When Your Pelvic Support System Fails," for more information on pelvic organ prolapse.

Figure 19: Incomplete Bladder Emptying with a Prolapse

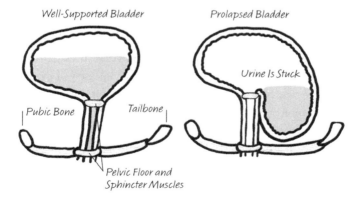

If your incomplete emptying is due to bladder or urethra prolapse or you simply feel that you need to push while peeing to get that last bit of urine out, try one or both of these techniques to help your bladder fully empty (instead of pushing to pee):

1. *Credé technique:* Once you feel like you're finished peeing (again, be sure you aren't pushing) and the urine stream has stopped, press below your belly button and lean forward. The compression of your hand will help to manually drain your bladder.

2. *Shimmy shake:* Yes, that's the real name; I made it up. Once you feel done (again, make sure you are not pushing), stand halfway up but keep your bum over the toilet and shake your hips side to side a few times. Then sit back down. This helps to reposition your bladder and urethra to get more urine out.

Feel free to get creative with these. I've had ladies do both of these twice through or use just one approach one time. I even had a woman take the shimmy shake to new heights by doing the shimmy shake sitting down and then standing up to march in place because she needed more motion than just shaking side to side to reposition her bladder to be fully empty. There is no wrong way; do what works best for you!

Peeing "Just in Case"

This behavior is rooted in us from childhood. How many of you remember your parents saying, "Come on, everyone, try to go to the bathroom before we leave"? We all do! This is called "just in case" peeing, where you don't really have to pee, but you go anyway, just in case you might have to go thirty minutes later when you're on the road or in a store—basically, at a less convenient time.

This must change! Here's why. As we discussed earlier, the bladder has receptors that can develop habits and memory. If you constantly pee "just in case" when your bladder isn't truly full by going when it's convenient (maybe even before you've had a first signal to pee), then over time your bladder can shrink, and it will give you a strong urge too soon.

Another reason to avoid "just in case" voiding is because it will lead to bladder behavioral issues. If you always go to the bathroom prior to leaving the house, before a work meeting, or every time you pass the bathroom, then over time you can develop strong urges to pee whenever you are in that situation. Also, if you do leave the house or start a meeting without peeing, then later when you think about it, you may get a sudden strong, uncontrollable urge based on your thoughts alone. At that point you may panic and enter the "fight or flight" state, because your bladder has established the memory of your routine and wants what it is used to.

Other common times that you may pee out of convenience include when you're in the shower or swimming in a body of water like the lake or ocean. (No peeing in the pool, please!) I'll be the first to admit I was guilty of this before I became a pelvic floor physical therapist. I'd like to blame my mom for my previous habit of peeing in the shower, although I've since forgiven her. I was potty trained to the sound of running water so I wouldn't be bashful to go. As a result, lucky me, every time I hear running water, I get an urge to pee. I can suppress it now, and it goes away quickly because I understand what is going on so I remain calm. However, before I understood any of this, whenever I heard water I'd be running to the bathroom, and, you guessed it, leaking. Not to mention that to take a shower, oh goodness, I didn't stand a chance. The bottom line is that if you pee in the shower or in a body of water, don't pee simply for the convenience factor. If you truly have to go, meaning it's the second or third signal, by all means go. I will caution you, though: if you're about to hop in the shower and do really have to go, then you should just sit on the toilet first and pee to avoid developing an associated reaction of whenever you're in the shower and hear the sound of running water, you pee.

I challenge you to begin changing your habits and to avoid peeing simply because it's convenient. Rather, wait until you truly do have to go. I also challenge you to let your children, grandchildren, or any other little ones in your life tell you when they need to pee. At a minimum, *offer* them a chance to pee versus *making* them try to pee "just in case."

Also, to spare them a lifelong struggle down the road, please don't turn on the faucet to help them start peeing. If they're bashful, let them sit alone, reassuring them that nobody can hear their bodily functions and that elimination is a normal process for everyone.

BLADDER IRRITANTS

The amount and type of fluids you drink will affect the signals your bladder gives you and how frequently you feel the need to pee. For example, caffeine, highly-acidic drinks like orange juice, carbonated drinks, and alcohols are known to be bladder irritants. (I know—all of the good stuff.) Have you ever noticed in the morning that after drinking your coffee, you have stronger urges or are peeing more frequently? If so, coffee may be an irritant to you. Even decaf, although it is not caffeinated, is still acidic and bothersome to some bladders.

So, what can you do about this while still enjoying the simple pleasures? I recommend using the sandwich approach, which I learned in elementary school. When giving constructive criticism, it's best to sandwich the feedback between two slices of praise: compliment, criticism, compliment. You can use the same idea for managing your bladder: drink a bladder-friendly fluid, then the irritant, then more bladder-friendly fluid. Table 4 contains a list of bladder-friendly fluids and irritants. If you forget to sandwich and you're already drinking an irritant, it's not too late! You can drink the bladder-friendly fluid between sips of the irritant: sip of water, sip of wine, sip of water, etc.

You might be wondering about cranberry juice and why it is not listed in the table. That's because it deserves a conversation. Cranberry juice is thought to decrease bacteria from adhering to the lining of the urinary tract and to promote an infection-resistant urine concentration.[15] It is important to note that cranberry juice can help *decrease risk of* urinary tract infections (UTIs), not *cure* them once you already have one. Recommendations remain up for debate on how often and how much you should drink to help prevent UTIs as well as what form of cranberry to take (e.g., juice, juice cocktail, or capsules). Additionally, cranberry juice is mildly acidic, so it can be irritating for some people's bladders and

Table 4: Bladder Fluid Guide

BLADDER-FRIENDLY FLUIDS	BLADDER IRRITANTS
• Pure water • Pure water with fruits, vegetables, or herbs added: berries, lemon, lime, cucumbers, basil, ginger, mint, rosemary • Mild juices: apple, grape, berry • Milk or milk alternatives • Decaf coffee and tea (however, although they are better than caffeinated versions, they can still be irritating)	• Caffeinated coffee and tea • Soda • Acidic juices: orange and tomato • Alcohol • Carbonated water • Drinks with artificial sweeteners

lead to bladder urgency and frequency. If you feel your bladder handles cranberry products well, then it is a bladder-friendly fluid and you can keep consuming it. If you find it to be irritating, consider avoiding it.

Let's talk about that morning cup of joe! Did you know your kidneys are constantly working and producing urine, even when you are not drinking? Think about when you wake up in the morning. One of the first things you do is pee, emptying a full bladder, even though you have not been drinking during the night. This is because of the kidneys—they are always working. When you wake up in the morning, you might notice that your pee is darker or has a stronger odor, which is because it is more concentrated. This is okay and normal! However, the concentration of this urine can be slightly irritating to your bladder overnight.

Why is that important? Well, let's say the first thing you drink in the morning is coffee. Drinking coffee on a slightly irritated bladder can really aggravate your bladder; it's screaming, "Get this out!" Instead, if the first thing you drink is a bladder-friendly fluid, like a glass of water, then you have a chance to calm your bladder prior to gulping down that coffee. Give it a try. It can certainly help minimize the strong urges and frequent peeing you may be experiencing after drinking your morning coffee. Along the same lines, drinking water with cocktails, beer, and wine will not only help your bladder but also lessen the potential headache in the morning! It's a win-win.

Here's another trick you can try if you have a Keurig machine. If you select the smallest pour, it has the least amount of water and is more concentrated. If you select the largest pour, there is more water, which means the coffee is diluted and less irritating. I still recommend that you drink a bladder-friendly fluid prior to your coffee, but the largest Keurig pour will help dilute the irritating coffee.

A good guide is to drink eight ounces of a bladder-friendly fluid (ideally, water) every ninety minutes or so. This ensures that your bladder is getting good fluid to keep it calm and to avoid a buildup of concentrated, acidic urine, which will irritate it. Some women are able to drink fluids right up until bedtime and still void only once during the night (or not at all), whereas others may need to cut fluids off about two hours prior to bedtime. Just don't cut off your fluid intake any sooner than that or you may end up with a buildup of concentrated, acidic urine in your bladder, which can cause irritation and result in excessive night time voiding.

Additionally, if you wake up during the night, resist the temptation of "just in case" voiding. Don't pee simply because you don't want to be woken up later. Instead, ask yourself if you *really* have to pee. Maybe you simply woke up because you are hot, cold, or uncomfortable; maybe your partner is snoring! If you are awake for any reason aside from needing to pee, do not pee unless you truly have to go. Resisting "just in case" voiding will help train your bladder to decrease nighttime voiding frequency and squash bad voiding habits. However, if your anxiety about waking up again to pee is so strong that you simply can't fall back asleep, then void if you must this time, but review this section again when you're feeling calmer and try to commit yourself to resisting temptation and forming better habits in the future.

Certain foods can irritate your bladder as well. Food irritants include tomato-based foods, spicy foods, citric fruits, and chocolate (again, the good stuff!). You can try the sandwich approach with food irritants as well: drink a bladder-friendly fluid before and after consuming the irritating food. If you forget to sandwich, sip a bladder-friendly fluid while you eat an irritating food.

Another strategy to reduce the effects of food and drink irritants is to use an over-the-counter product called Prelief, which reduces the acidity of food and drinks, causing less irritation to the bladder.[16] It is available in a tablet or power form; consult your healthcare provider to see if this could be a good option for you.

URGENCY AND FREQUENCY

Some of you may also experience "close calls" by having strong and/or frequent urges to pee. Let's nip this situation in the "butt" before it develops into leaking! Remember that your bladder has receptors, and with urgency and frequency, you essentially need to work on reprograming your bladder to stop sending an early, urgent signal to pee. Of note, you may experience urgency and frequency in addition to leaking. If that is the case, make sure you read the "Urinary Incontinence" section that is next.

Taking specific steps to control your fluid intake, spacing, and pacing are crucial for this to work. We already talked about bladder irritants, and although the idea of drinking coffee, seltzer, and wine all day may sound great, you must sandwich these irritants with water and drink water throughout the day! There are two different approaches you can try for water intake:

1. Drink eight, eight-ounce glasses of water a day.
2. Drink half your body weight in ounces of water a day.

Everyone is different, and for some people, the amount of fluid they would need to drink to equal half of their body weight would just be too much. I suggest trying both options to see what works for you; maybe you'll find that your best match falls somewhere in the middle of what each strategy recommends.

Regarding spacing and pacing of fluid, a good goal is to drink eight ounces of water about every ninety minutes or so. This will keep a consistent flow of friendly fluids in your bladder. However, you should also be aware of the fact that if you quickly drink more than eight ounces of any fluid, this can aggravate your bladder because you're asking it to stretch too quickly, leading to a strong urge and the need to pee frequently.

Let's pause for just a minute here, because I bet some of you ladies are thinking I must have it backward. How can I be asking you to constantly drink water throughout the day if you're trying to decrease bladder urgency and frequency? Wouldn't drinking less water make more sense? Let's bust this myth right here and now. Drinking only small amounts of water does not work because your kidneys are constantly producing urine regardless of your intake. We've already talked about how drinking coffee first thing in the morning means that you are drinking an irritant on top of an already irritated bladder (due to the concentrated urine that accumulated in the bladder all night). The same concept applies during the day. Your kidneys are constantly producing urine, so if you're not drinking fluids, especially bladder-friendly fluids like water, then during the day the concentrated urine can aggravate your bladder, leading to . . . you guessed it: urgency, frequency, and—potentially—even leaking. Some of you might still be thinking my approach won't work, especially if you feel that every time you drink water, you need to pee. This could be because you are drinking too much water too quickly. If you drink water "just to get it over with" and chug a glass every few hours, then your bladder will have to stretch too quickly and it will still give you a strong urge to go. This is why pacing and spacing of fluids is so important! Additionally, if you drink ice-cold water, it may irritate your bladder. Try drinking water that is at room temperature to see if that helps decrease any strong urge you feel after drinking water.

There are two strategies you can use to help your bladder return to its normal size so it can better fill and store urine. As you review these strategies, note that they will work only if you are drinking enough water, appropriately spaced throughout the day. These strategies will also help reset your bladder receptors back to normal to decrease urgency and frequency. Here they are:

1. *Urge signaling:* This method allows you to gradually build your bladder's tolerance to holding urine. With urge signaling, you want to suppress the first urge to pee so that you pee only on the second or third signal instead. (See the earlier section "How the Bladder Works," for specifics on each of the three signals.)

    Here's how it might look. All of a sudden (maybe after you drink your coffee or hear running water), you get a strong urge to pee. Suppress this urge by using your mantras, crossing your legs (a discussion on why this works is ahead!), and distracting yourself. Remember, you must stay calm for the urge to pass. Once it has passed, continue with what you were doing when you felt the first urge. Later, when you feel a second urge creeping up on you, repeat this process again. At that point, you can either go to the bathroom or, if you suppressed the urge and feel well enough in control, wait to go until the third urge. Even if you're only able to suppress the first urge for a few minutes before needing to pee on the second signal, that is okay! The point is that you are demonstrating to your bladder that *you* are in control and will pee when *you* decide it is time to go, not when your bladder prompts you.

2. *Timed voiding:* If the urge signal program isn't working for you, try this method next. You now know that normal voiding occurs every two to four hours. If you're following a different, erratic schedule, such as voiding every thirty minutes in the morning but not for another six hours after that, then your bladder can get very confused.

    With timed voiding, you are mindful of the time between each void, picking a time frame you feel you can be successful with. In the morning, maybe instead of going every thirty minutes, you wait forty-five minutes or an hour. Midday, if it's been more than four hours since you last peed, go to the bathroom. If you're not getting an urge to pee, it could be that you're not drinking your fluids appropriately. Be very mindful of your fluid intake, and make sure you're evenly pacing your fluids throughout the day to help with this bladder retraining. The goal of timed voiding is to help your bladder restore its signal program so then you can switch to the urge-signaling program mentioned earlier. Once you are able to pee at your selected timed voiding interval without leaking for a full day, try lengthening the time between intervals by ten minutes at a stretch. By doing this, you should start to notice a more normal voiding schedule of every two to four hours.

With both urge signaling and timed voiding, the goal is to build up your bladder's ability to store urine and provide appropriate signals to pee without leaking so you can make it calmly to the bathroom. Both programs can be intertwined, setting a timed voiding goal and using the urge-signaling program to avoid going too early.

URINARY INCONTINENCE

Leaking urine, known as incontinence, is not normal. It also should not be an acceptable symptom of aging, whether you've ever given birth or not. This is so important, I'll say it again: *it is not normal.* You should not have to wear "bladder leak underwear" or liners for the rest of your life; nor should you need to know where all of the public bathrooms are like your life depends on it. My blood boils when I see commercials of women dancing around appearing delighted to be wearing bladder leak underwear as if it's an acceptable normalcy. Hello! There *is* a solution, and you can get help with physical therapy.

Now is when we have an important chat about Kegels—I know you've been waiting for it! Urinary incontinence can present itself whether you have weak or tight pelvic floor muscles, but the solution is different in each case. The quick explanation for this goes as follows: If your pelvic floor muscles are already tight, then they will not be able to squeeze to engage any further when you are trying to hold back urine. This means that Kegels will only make the problem worse. On the other hand, if your pelvic floor muscles are weak, then they will lack the strength to squeeze to engage to close the urethral opening. In this case, Kegels can help. Consequently, it is imperative for you to determine which route you need—lengthening or strengthening. This is thoroughly covered in chapter 7, "To Lengthen or Strengthen." In the meantime, let's take a closer look at just what urinary incontinence is and how it can be classified.

Stress Urinary Incontinence (SUI)

Stress urinary incontinence (SUI) happens when there is stress placed on your bladder from an increase in abdominal pressure, without the proper support from your pelvic floor muscles. SUI commonly occurs with coughing, sneezing, laughing, exercise, and/or lifting.

Normally, your pelvic floor muscles and core muscles will automatically squeeze to engage right before you cough, sneeze, laugh, lift, or do any task that results in increased abdominal pressure. This automatic squeeze provides support to your internal organs by lifting your bladder and closing the urethra so that the force produced by your pelvic floor muscles and core muscles is greater than the force produced in abdominal pressure from the task. This results in a counterbrace and prevents leaking. Then, when your body has completed the task, your pelvic floor muscles and core muscles should automatically relax so they do not stay tensed.

This essential physical response is called "the knack" simply because our bodies have the automatic knack for doing it. However, sometimes women lose this counterbrace reflex, so they are more prone to leaking. Fortunately, this reflex is trainable, and you can get it back with practice. Here's how it works, using sneezing as an example: in the split second before you sneeze, *squeeze!*

You should use this simple, protective step with any task that increases abdominal pressure. The biggest challenge is remembering to do

Figure 20: Increased Abdominal Pressure on the Bladder Without and With the Knack

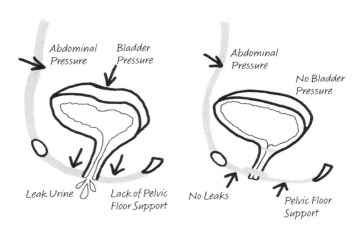

it! Figure 20 shows how the bladder responds with increased abdominal pressure without and with the knack.

Another factor contributing to stress urinary incontinence is having a hysterectomy, or the removal of your uterus. The uterus sits behind the bladder, as shown in figure 21, and when it is removed, your body does not hold its place. Rather, the surrounding organs fill in, as shown in figure 22. Unfortunately, uterus, you don't get a memorial statue. Therefore, the bladder will lose its backstop, the uterus, and undergo more movement with coughing, sneezing, laughing, and lifting. The knack can certainly help by providing more support to the bladder from the pelvic floor muscles, but sometimes women may need to be fitted for a pessary. As we discussed in chapter 2, "When Your Pelvic Support System Fails," a pessary is an elastic or rigid device that is inserted into the vagina. In this case, the pessary takes up space where the uterus previously was, which in turn provides support to the bladder to help decrease SUI. This is something your gynecologist can help you with.

Figure 21: The Pelvic Organs

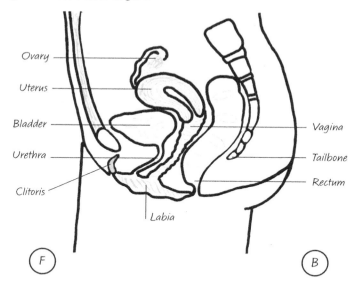

Ovary

Uterus

Bladder

Urethra

Clitoris

Labia

Vagina

Tailbone

Rectum

F

B

Figure 22: The Pelvic Organs Without the Uterus

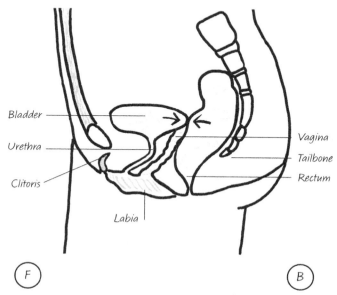

Bladder

Urethra

Clitoris

Labia

Vagina

Tailbone

Rectum

F

B

Chronic coughing can also contribute to SUI. Excessive coughing with a bad cold, smoking, or chronic obstructive pulmonary disease places excessive demand on your pelvic floor to support the organs against an increase in abdominal pressure. This is especially true if you are not doing the knack while coughing. If you are doing the knack but you are still leaking, then you must identify the state of your pelvic floor muscles (either tense or weak) and address that issue appropriately. A pelvic floor physical therapist will help guide you through this diagnosis and treatment. Also see chapter 7, "To Lengthen or Strengthen," for more information.

Urge Urinary Incontinence (UUI)

Urge urinary incontinence (UUI) occurs when you have a really strong urge to pee and cannot hold it. Your bladder sends a demandingly strong signal that you have to go NOW, you rush (trying to outrun your bladder), and then you leak. As mentioned previously, this could stem from irritating fluids, lack of good fluids, poor fluid spacing, and/or poorly trained behaviors that have led to inappropriate bladder contractions. Although the state of your pelvic floor muscles (tense or weak) may play a role, more often than not you can eliminate UUI by addressing your bad bladder habits.

Bad bladder habits can lead to UUI. As we've discussed already, if you pee "just in case" when you are about to leave the house, you will start getting a strong urge to pee *every* time you are about to leave the house, and this can then lead to leaking (UUI). Likewise, if you rush to the bathroom right when you get home because of a sudden urge (a situation called "key in the door syndrome"), it is nearly impossible to gain control of the urge, causing you to leak as you try to make it to the bathroom (UUI).

To address this issue, use the techniques discussed in the "Feeling Out of Control" section earlier in this chapter. Additionally, you can use the following tricks to try to suppress, or at least decrease, the strong urge to pee:

- *Calf raises:* The calf muscles and pelvic floor muscles share a nerve root, which means that the nerve that supplies your calf muscle starts from the same spot as the nerve that supplies your pelvic floor muscles. Therefore, when you do a calf raise (which is also known as a heel raise) to squeeze the calf muscles, also think about squeezing your pelvic floor muscles. The calf raise can automatically assist with generating a stronger pelvic floor muscle squeeze. We know through Bradly's Loop (our reciprocal relationship reflex) that when we are squeezing our pelvic floor the bladder relaxes, decreasing the strong urge to pee. To do a heel raise, lift your heels up off the ground when you are standing or sitting so your weight is on the balls of your feet; you will feel your calf muscles squeezing. Repeat as many times as needed to decrease the urgent need to pee.
- *Crossing your legs:* This engages your groin muscles, the adductor group, which are "helper muscles" to the pelvic floor muscles. When you cross your legs and engage your groin muscles, you get a stronger pelvic floor muscle squeeze. Like calf raises, this helps to calm the bladder urge through Bradly's Loop, and crossing your legs also helps to close the urethra. I'm sure you've seen this before with children: they're crossing their legs, squirming around, and saying they have to pee!

Mixed Urinary Incontinence (MUI)

MUI occurs when you experience both SUI and UUI. Usually, one is worse than the other and one began prior to the other. Regardless, it is important to address both.

Overflow and Insensible Incontinence

There are two more types of incontinence that are worth a quick discussion because pelvic floor physical therapy can help with each.

Overflow incontinence occurs when you aren't aware of your bladder's signals as it fills, so it becomes too full to stretch anymore.

Then it "overflows" and urine leaks out. Women with overflow incontinence usually experience other symptoms too, including some of the following:

- Incomplete bladder emptying
- Difficulty starting the urine stream
- Decreased voiding volume when peeing (you are unable to have a stream that lasts for a count of 10 "Mississippis")
- A weak urine stream
- A start-and-stop urine stream
- Frequent urinary tract infections

There are several reasons that overflow incontinence could be happening. For example, it may occur with a pelvic organ prolapse, scar tissue around the urethra, or bladder stones—anything that may block the urine's path from the bladder from exiting through the urethra. Overflow incontinence may also be due to signaling issues between the brain, spinal cord, bladder, nerves, and muscles, and it usually requires further investigation to identify the causes and solutions.

When insensible urinary incontinence occurs, you can't tell that the leakage is actually happening. Instead, you later realize that your underwear or panty liner is wet. Three steps are needed to help you identify the causes and solutions for this type of incontinence:

1. Close tracking of fluid intake and voiding habits
2. Understanding how the bladder works
3. Ensuring that you are drinking good fluids evenly spaced throughout the day

Pelvic floor physical therapy is strongly recommended for both overflow and insensible incontinence because there are several variables to consider. In the meantime, try implementing the strategies mentioned throughout this chapter so that you understand your bladder's signals, what normal voiding frequency is, and how and when to drink enough good fluids throughout the day.

Eliminating Safety Nets

No matter which type of incontinence you experience, it is important to wean from pads, liners, and bladder leak underwear if you are using them on a regular basis. If you do need pads or liners as a temporary measure, be sure the products you choose are designed for incontinence versus for periods, because the two types are made of different material and have different mechanisms for wicking away urine versus blood.

Pads, liners, and bladder leak underwear act as safety nets, and whether you are conscious of it or not, you may not try as hard to make it to the bathroom because of this safety net. In other words, you may start thinking, "It's okay if I leak a little; the pad will catch it." No, it's not okay! Instead, build up your confidence by using the strategies mentioned throughout this chapter. Then try going pad-less in your home, for just an hour or two. Your home is the safest environment to ditch the pad, because if you do leak, you have a change of clothes and a private bathroom to clean up in! From here, you will slowly build up your ability to completely go pad-free at home.

For the next step, run a short errand out of your house without a pad—and don't think about peeing "just in case" prior to leaving the house, either! You might be reading this with your eyes as big as saucers, thinking I'm insane. Believe me, you can do it, even if this goal takes you a month or even several months to reach. Don't get too far ahead of yourself; take this one step at a time. After all, you're trying to change behaviors and habits that may have been present for years. When you're ready to run your short errand, pick someplace with a public bathroom that's easy to access, like the grocery store or the library. Before you leave, tell yourself that if you need to, you can pee once you get there *if* you have to; give yourself this mental checkpoint of safety. You can also carry a pad and a change of underwear in your purse if that makes you feel more comfortable.

Once you've mastered the pad-less short errand, leave the pad off for longer periods of time: running a longer errand, a half day at work, visiting a friend, etc. To avoid the "fight or flight" nervous system state, you must feel confident and safe to do this, though, so take your time, be patient and kind to yourself with your progress, and celebrate the small successes you achieve! In time, you will find that you become less obsessive about having a pad on. On that first day you get home and realize you went all day without a pad, you'll feel great about your accomplishments—and your lady parts will thank you for being able to breathe!

URINARY TRACT INFECTIONS

I know it may seem elementary to include information on urinary tract infections (UTIs), because most of us understand what this might feel like. But, did you know a UTI could happen in the kidneys, the ureters, the bladder, or the urethra? In fact, they can occur anywhere along the entire urinary tract, which is shown in figure 23.

Figure 23: The Urinary Tract System

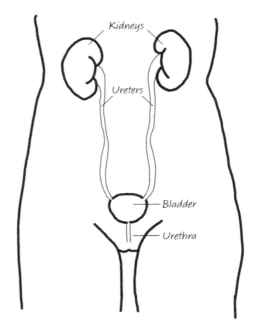

Symptoms include pain or burning when peeing, strong urges to pee, and/or blood in the urine. Uncommon symptoms can include back or lower abdominal pain and pressure; feeling fatigued, shaky, confused, and weak; or having a fever. These symptoms can present all together or individually. I am including the uncommon symptoms because I have seen them firsthand. One of my physical therapy patients, a sweet woman I'll call Jane, was referred to me by her doctor with complaints of low back pain. She had no other bladder symptoms, although sometimes she needed to pee frequently. As we progressed with the physical therapy, Jane was not getting better, and I noticed she often seemed spacey and confused. I sent her back to her doctor because something just did not seem right. In this case, she had none of the typical symptoms, but upon further evaluation she did indeed have a UTI. Once it was treated, her back pain and confusion went away.

If you feel you have a UTI, be sure your doctor tests your urine. Sometimes, pelvic pain diagnoses or infections such as bacterial vaginosis or interstitial cystitis can mimic symptoms of a UTI. If your UTI testing is negative, demand further investigation to get the answers and treatment you need.

Women get UTIs more frequently than men do because our urethra is shorter, making it easier for bacteria to get into the bladder. Our urethral opening is also closer to the vaginal and rectal openings, making it easier for bacteria to enter. All the more important to wipe front to back!

CHAPTER FIVE

Bowel Health

"Roses are red, violets are blue,
raise up your knees whenever you poo!"

—Unknown

Until I started my work as a physical therapist, I never knew it was possible to become so fascinated with the bowels and stool, more commonly known as poop. Your stool provides valuable information about your diet and about your pelvic floor. When you're done reading this chapter, you will look in the toilet at your poop every single time, I just know it, because it's that engrossing—not to be confused with, "Ew, gross!"

The bowels are part of the digestive process, which actually starts at the other end of the tube: your mouth. I highly recommend reading the book *Gut: The Inside Story of Our Body's Most Underrated Organ* by Giulia Enders for a great read on this entire process.[17] For the sake of this guide, we are going to review briefly the anatomy of the digestive system with a focus on the large intestine onward. Let's "gut" started!

ANATOMY

Digestion begins at your mouth. As soon as you see or smell food, your salivary glands turn on, producing more saliva to help break down your food. When you smell something delicious, does your mouth start watering? I know I'm not the only one! Obviously, chewing breaks down food as well, and it stimulates the gastrocolic reflex. Have you ever eaten a meal and, shortly thereafter, had a bowel movement? That is the gastrocolic reflex: the act of chewing and eating food stimulates your entire digestive tract, pushing its contents along, resulting in a bowel movement.

After chewing, food then travels to the stomach, where it is churned prior to being pushed along to the small intestine. Here, in the small intestine, is where the majority of nutrients are broken down and absorbed. The small intestine next joins the large intestine through a one-way valve known as the ileocecal valve. This valve monitors passage of nutrients, fluid, and bacteria from the small to the large intestine. Sometimes, this valve can get stuck open or closed. If that occurs, a pelvic floor physical therapist can help identify issues within the ileocecal valve with diet, lifestyle changes (such as stress reduction), and massage to the valve to ensure that it functions optimally. Once the food gets through the valve, it is moved along to the large intestine, and here is where we delve in.

The large intestine, also known as the colon, is responsible for further absorbing water and the remaining nutrients that the small intestine did not absorb. It is also acts as a transit system to eliminate waste, also known as poop. The large intestine starts at the right lower quadrant of your abdomen, which is to the right side of your belly button. It then travels up, across your abdomen under your rib cage, and down to the left lower quadrant, or the left side of your belly button. Here, it meets the sigmoid colon joining the rectum and the anus—then it's "Hello, toilet bowl." Take a look at figure 24.

Of note, your appendix is situated in your right lower quadrant, to the right of your belly button. To check for appendicitis, you can perform a Rebound Tenderness Test. Press on the right side of your belly halfway between your belly button and pelvic bone. When you release the pressure, if your pain gets worse it's a positive test, which means you should seek medical attention immediately for further investigation because your appendix could rupture. I've been there, and it's not fun!

Figure 24: The Entire Digestive Tract

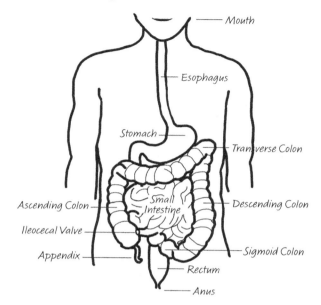

Mouth

Esophagus

Stomach

Transverse Colon

Small Intestine

Ascending Colon

Descending Colon

Ileocecal Valve

Appendix

Sigmoid Colon

Rectum

Anus

HOW THE BOWELS WORK

We know that the large intestine is responsible for absorbing the remaining water and nutrients from your food, a process that aids in the formation of your poop. The large intestine pushes stool along via mass movements, which is also called peristalsis. Imagine peristalsis as a wave-like motion occurring throughout your large intestine.

Once poop enters the rectum, flaps known as Folds of Houston help slow down your poop's descent. This is so you aren't quickly overwhelmed with the urge to have a bowel movement. After the rectum comes the anus, which is comprised of two muscles: the internal anal sphincter and the external anal sphincter. These are circular muscles that further help control your poop's descent. Figure 25 shows each of these parts in the rectum.

Figure 25: The Rectum

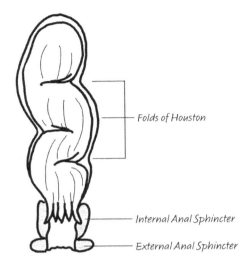

Folds of Houston

Internal Anal Sphincter

External Anal Sphincter

The next part is actually really cool! You have a reflex called the Recto-Anal Inhibitory Reflex (RAIR), also known as the "sampling reflex." The internal anal sphincter muscle relaxes just a little bit, allowing a small sample of solid stool, liquid stool, or gas to pass toward the opening to let your body sense what is coming. (See figures 26, 27, and 28.)

If the sample is gas and the circumstances are appropriate, let it rip. If the sample is solid stool or liquid stool (or gas at an inappropriate time), then the outer sphincter muscle will squeeze so nothing escapes. This is called the Recto-Anal Contractile Reflex (RACR), because your muscle contracts to hold back the sample. You then know that it's time to make a plan to get to the bathroom. Who knew our bodies were so smart?

If this last part of your bowels (especially the anal sphincter muscles, which are part of the pelvic floor muscles) cannot detect "samples" or are too tight or weak, then you can experience problems like constipation, diarrhea, or fecal incontinence. Before we delve into deeper details, keep in mind that there are numerous causes to bowel dysfunction: side effects from medications, emotions such as stress and anxiety, and dietary

Figure 26: A Solid Stool Sample

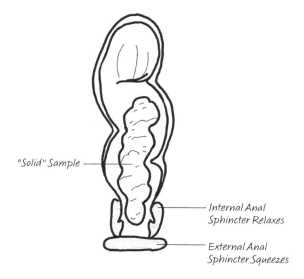

"Solid" Sample

Internal Anal
Sphincter Relaxes

External Anal
Sphincter Squeezes

Figure 27: A Liquid Stool Sample

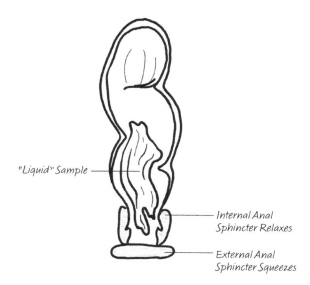

"Liquid" Sample

Internal Anal
Sphincter Relaxes

External Anal
Sphincter Squeezes

Figure 28: A Gas Sample

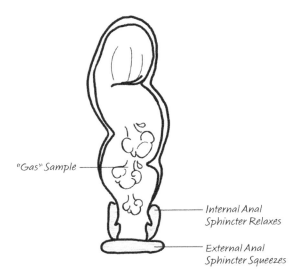

"Gas" Sample

Internal Anal
Sphincter Relaxes

External Anal
Sphincter Squeezes

intolerances. It usually requires a team approach from your healthcare providers to identify these causes, but rest assured, a pelvic floor physical therapist will help guide you throughout your course of treatment!

WHAT IS NORMAL

Unlike the bladder, which is designed to hold and store, the bowels are designed for transit, movement, and elimination. When you have an urge to poop, you should be making a plan to do so sooner rather than later. You might be thinking, "Can't it wait until I'm in the comfort of my home versus at work or out in public?" No, it can't. And, you know what? Everyone poops. If someone from the next restroom stall hears you deposit with a plunk in the toilet or pass gas, who cares? We all do it! More important, here's why it can't wait: your poop is a waste product, so if you ignore the urge, your body continues to absorb what you don't need and dries it out. This ultimately causes it to be more difficult for you to poop later, and you may start to feel sluggish and bloated.

Bowel Movement Frequency

So, how often should you poop? Well, frequency of bowel movements vary from person to person, with the normal range anywhere from three times per day to three times per week. Three times a day may seem like a lot, but as previously explained, the gastrocolic reflex pushes contents along the digestive tract. So, every time you eat a meal, you might have the urge to have a bowel movement . . . what goes in eventually makes its way out after your body takes what it needs. You must correlate the frequency of your bowel movements with your symptoms, such as feeling bloated, incomplete bowel emptying, or difficulty passing stool. As unlikely as it may seem, someone can still be constipated despite having a bowel movement every day.

Bowel Movement Shape and Consistency

Basically, what does your poop look like? Believe it or not, there's a chart for classifying our poop to help us understand if we are experiencing constipation or diarrhea. It's called the Bristol Stool Chart, and you can check it out in figure 29. This chart can help you normalize the language you use to talk about the "types" of poop you have and where you're at, ranging from constipation (Type 1) to diarrhea (Type 7). Later in this chapter we will discuss what you can do if you're on either end of the spectrum.

The Bristol Stool Chart does a nice job at depicting stool shape, but it does not touch on the issue of pencil-thin stool. Pencil-thin stool can be indicative of tension within your pelvic floor muscles. If your pelvic floor muscles cannot fully relax, then there is a smaller opening for stool to pass through, which can lead to a pencil-like appearance. Stool that looks like this can be of hard consistency (Type 2) to soft, normal consistency (Type 4), but usually it will be soft (Type 4). For further information on how to address tight pelvic floor muscles, please refer to page 97.

Figure 29: The Bristol Stool Chart

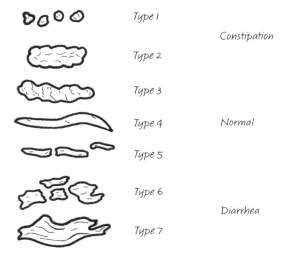

Type 1

Type 2   Constipation

Type 3

Type 4   Normal

Type 5

Type 6

Type 7   Diarrhea

Please note, you should seek medical attention if you experience any of the following symptoms:

- Bright-red or dark-black coloring to your stool, especially if it also has a pencil-thin appearance
- A change in your bowel movement frequency
- Abdominal pain
- Unexplained weight loss or weight gain
- Symptoms of fatigue

Your doctor will likely order a colonoscopy to investigate, as these can be signs and symptoms of colon cancer and other issues, such as Crohn's Disease.

Bowel Movement Color

The last detail we need to talk about is stool color. Brown to greenish-brown poop is considered normal; the color is the result of precise interactions between the entire digestive tract. There are several variations of what color your stool could be. Let's take a look:

Black: This can suggest bleeding along the gastrointestinal tract, especially if your poop looks like coffee grounds. If you experience black, coffee-ground-like stool, seek medical attention immediately.

Green: If you've eaten an abundance of green foods like spinach or kale, you may have green poop. Green-colored stool can also be a result of stool moving too fast through the digestive process, decreasing the amount of nutrients actually absorbed and contributing to loose stool (Type 6 and Type 7). When this happens, bile (a fluid that aids in digestion produced by the liver and stored in the gallbladder) is not broken down and contributes to the green color. If you consistently have loose green stool, consult a gastrointestinal doctor.

Red: Hemorrhoids can cause a small amount of red color in your stool, from blood; this is usually nothing to worry about. (Check out the "Hemorrhoids" section in this chapter.) However, if you experience a medium to large amount of red color in your stool, this can be indicative of a gastrointestinal bleed and requires immediate medical attention. This is especially true if you have not consumed red foods such as beets, red berries, tomato juice, or beet juice.

Orange: Usually, orange stool is a result of eating excessive amounts of carrots, squash, and sweet potatoes, all of which contain beta-carotene, giving the foods themselves the orange color. However, if you experience orange stool without having eaten orange-colored foods, it can indicate an issue with the bile of your digestive system and requires a consult with a gastrointestinal doctor.

Yellow: Usually yellow-colored stool is accompanied by a greasy, fatty-like appearance too. This is indicative of too much fat in your stool from your body's decreased ability to absorb fat. If you notice this occurring frequently, consult a gastrointestinal doctor.

CONSTIPATION

There is an actual objective measure to determine if you're constipated. It's called Rome Criteria IV: Constipation. A group of health professionals actually meet in Rome every six to ten years to talk about the bowels, and they publish new criteria after every meeting. I'd love to go to Rome and discuss bowel health!

If you're ever wondering if you're truly constipated, glance over my summary of Rome Criteria IV: Constipation:[18]

- Your symptoms began at least six months ago but have been present for at least the last three months.
- You rarely have loose stools.
- You do not meet the qualifications for irritable bowel syndrome (IBS), which are recurrent abdominal pain more than one day per week in the last three months and two or more of the following criteria: a bowel movement that either increases or decreases pain; a change in bowel movement frequency; a change in stool type. For more on this topic, refer to the IBS section within this chapter.
- You have more than two of the following at least 25 percent of the time:
  - » You experience incomplete bowel emptying.
  - » You use manual maneuvers to eliminate, such as bowel splinting.
  - » You have less than three *spontaneous* bowel movements a week.
  - » You feel obstructed evacuation, or blockage, when trying to have a bowel movement.
  - » Your stools qualify as Type 1 or 2 on the Bristol Stool Chart (hard lumps).
  - » You strain to empty.

There can be various reasons you may be experiencing constipation. Seeing a pelvic floor physical therapist can help identify your specific needs.

Whether you meet the criteria for constipation or simply struggle with feeling constipated every now and then, you can try the following strategies.

Increasing Water Consumption

In chapter 4, "Bladder Health," you learned how important it is to consistently drink water throughout the day. Well, this can also help you have better bowel movements because it will soften your stool! Try to consistently drink eight ounces of water about every two hours.

Heeding the Urge to Go

If you feel an urge to poop, try to go sooner rather than later. Holding it back will cause your stool to become harder and dryer, ultimately making it more difficult to pass. I know how annoying or uncomfortable it can be to interrupt your work day to use the public bathroom and poop. However, your bowels will thank you in the long run!

Eating Insoluble Fiber

Add more insoluble fiber to your diet. Insoluble fiber helps move hard, dry stool through your large intestine. This raises two questions: First, what are some good sources of insoluble fiber? Second, should people use over-the-counter supplements like laxatives or stool softeners? Table 5 shows some sources of insoluble fiber.

Table 5: Sources of Insoluble Fiber to Move Stool

Fruits: apples, berries, cherries, grapes, melon, nectarines, peaches, pears, pineapple, prunes, raisins
Juice: apple, pear, prune
Nuts and seeds: almonds, chia seeds, flax seeds, sunflower seeds, walnuts
Vegetables: bell peppers, broccoli, Brussel sprouts, cauliflower, celery, corn, cucumber, green beans, lettuce greens, peas, spinach, tomatoes
Other sources: popcorn, whole grains, whole wheat

As a general approach, I suggest you start with adding insoluble fiber through your food intake. If that doesn't work and the other strategies mentioned in this section don't help either, consult your doctor about the best over-the-counter supplement for you. Table 6 offers details about some of the most common products available.

Table 6: Supplements to Promote Bowel Movements

SUPPLEMENT	HOW IT WORKS
MiraLAX	Draws water into the colon to soften stool but does not change (e.g., speed up or slow down) colon transit time.
Metamucil, Psyllium Husk, Citrucel, Benefiber	Draws water into the colon, softens stool, and adds bulk to stool in an attempt to stimulate a normal bowel movement.
Milk of Magnesia	Draws water into the colon to soften stool, and increases colon transit time, which means that stool is moved through the colon more quickly.
Senna, Ex-Lax	Irritates the lining of the colon to stimulate a bowel movement.
Dulcolax	Enables additional water and fats to be incorporated into the stool, softening the stool and making it easier to move through the colon.

Exercising

Generally speaking, this saying is true: when you move, your bowels move. When you are inactive, your bowels are inactive. Aim to get some form of activity for thirty minutes a day. This doesn't have to be anything special; it can be something as simple as going for a walk or taking the stairs versus the elevator all day at work.

In addition to staying active, you can perform stretching. Because the large intestine moves throughout the abdominal wall, tight surrounding muscles can limit its ability to push poop along. Specifically, you should stretch your psoas and quadratus lumborum (QL) muscles by doing a sixty-second hold two or three times a day. Here are descriptions and illustrations of these two stretches.

Psoas stretch (figure 30): Kneel so your right knee is on a pillow and your left foot is planted in front of you. Keep your hips pointing straight ahead and your chest tall and straight. Reach your right arm overhead, feeling a stretch through the front of your right hip and into the right side of your trunk. Hold for sixty seconds and then switch knees and repeat the stretch on your left side. You will feel the second stretch on your left hip and into the left side of your trunk.

Figure 30: Psoas Stretch

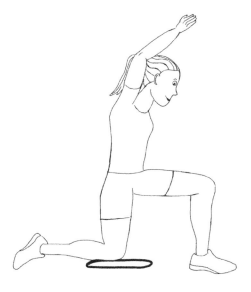

Quadratus lumborum stretch (figure 31): Lay on your left side with your right knee bent over your straight left leg. Prop up your trunk with your left arm, curving your trunk in the shape of the letter C away from the ground. Keep your hips perfectly stacked on top of each other. You will feel a stretch through the left side of your trunk. Hold for sixty seconds and then reverse the directions to repeat lying on your right side.

Figure 31: Quadratus Lumborum Stretch

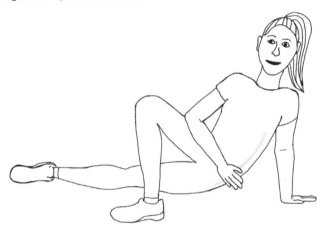

Massaging Abdominal Scar Tissue

If you've had any sort of abdominal surgery, scar tissue from the surgery may be blocking your large intestine's ability to push stool along. Scar tissue restrictions from a c-section or from the removal of any abdominal organ, like your appendix or gallbladder, are examples. If you do have scar tissue, just start rubbing it; there is no wrong way to perform a scar massage. I suggest using two fingers with moderate pressure in a circular direction clockwise and counterclockwise, vertical, diagonal, horizontal, or in zig-zag patterns. Massage the scar for five to ten minutes a day to aid in breaking up any restrictions.

Drinking Warm Liquids and Massaging Your Colon

Warm liquids stimulate the bowels and help with peristalsis, the movement of stool through the colon. This approach is particularly effective when you follow this step with a colon massage, which manually helps stimulate movement to push stool along. A glass of hot water with lemon is a great option; hot tea also works well. After you have the warm drink, perform the colon massage. I know this sounds weird, but it really can help!

This massage is best done lying flat on your back so your abdominal muscles are relaxed. You can also do it on the toilet, but it may not be as effective. For the massage, refer to figure 32. Start by doing ten circular motions, using a flat hand, starting at spot 5 on your left, then repeat the circular motions to spot 4, spot 3, spot 2, and lastly to spot 1 on your right. Next, use gentle, consistent pressure with a flat hand to sweep along the large intestine's path from spot 1 to spot 5. Repeat for ten sweeps.

Figure 32: Colon Massage Points

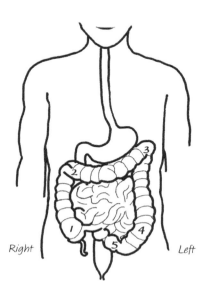

So, just how does this silly-sounding colon massage work? Think of the colon as the road and your poop as the cars. Ladies, when you are constipated, you have one bad traffic jam going on. And just like in a traffic jam, the lead car—which in this case is the poop closest to your anus in spot 5—has to move first to get everything moving again.

As you are doing this, you may hear gurgling noises or even feel light movement. Both are good—it means your body is responding. After the massage, you should go to the bathroom to try to have a bowel movement. In the next section we'll discuss just how to sit on the toilet.

You might be wondering if you should actually sit on the toilet after the colon massage even if you don't have an urge. The answer is yes, because the bowels are trainable and the act of sitting and relaxing (not straining) on the toilet can help stimulate your bowels!

Using Good Toilet Posture

To put it simply, good toilet posture involves sitting on the toilet with your knees elevated above your hips when you poo. This relaxed, squat-like position puts slack on the muscle that slings around the rectum, the puborectalis muscle, as seen in figure 33.

When this muscle is put on slack (think of the muscle as having more flexibility), your poop has more room to move through the rectum, making it easier to pass. You still must sit on the toilet seat, though; hovering will cause your pelvic floor muscles to be tense, which will block your poop's exit. This type of positioning is especially helpful during a bout of constipation, but for sake of ease, it can be used for every bowel movement even if you are not constipated.

To best achieve the position of your knees above your hips, use a stack of books, a foam roller, your trash can flipped on its side, a Squatty Potty (a specially designed bathroom footstool), a box, or anything else you can find to put your feet on. Next, spread your feet and knees apart to further open and relax the pelvic floor muscles. Keep your spine long (don't slouch!), and then lean forward, placing your elbows on your knees. This ensures that your tailbone is out of the way to open the back half of your bum further yet to help your poop pass more easily. Try to

Figure 33: Slacked Puborectalis Muscle

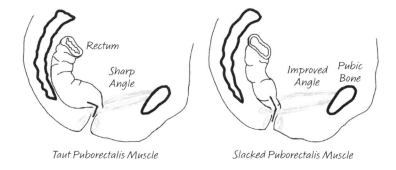

Taut Puborectalis Muscle   Slacked Puborectalis Muscle

Figure 34: Toilet Posture

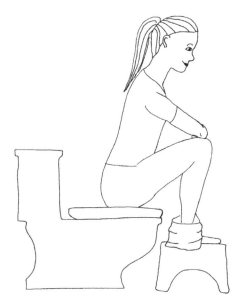

achieve the position shown in Figure 34.

Now perhaps you might be wondering what to do in a public restroom where there isn't something to place your feet on. A great alternative is to raise your heels so the weight of your legs are on the balls of your feet. This will at least get your knees in the right direction relative to your hips! You should still place your elbows on your knees, avoiding slouching so your spine is long and tall.

Now that you know how to achieve an optimal position, we need to talk about pushing. No more of the eyes-bulging-out-of-your head, breath-holding, grunting pushing. This type of straining places too much downward pressure on your pelvic floor, and it can contribute to developing a prolapse or worsen any symptoms of one. If you have a rectal prolapse or experience incomplete bowel emptying, you may benefit from rectal splinting. (Refer to page 16 and figure 12: Splinting for Rectal Prolapse for review on this topic.)

So, instead of straining and holding your breath (the Valsalva maneuver we discussed earlier in the book), you should breathe out while giving a *gentle* push, which is mostly generated by your exhale. Making sounds like "Shhhh," "Hmm," or "Haaa"—or even pretending to blow out candles while exhaling—can help. Play around with which breath sound works the best for you; it should be one that still allows you to relax through the back half of your bum.

Improving Your Coordination

To have a bowel movement, your pelvic floor muscles need to relax and lengthen. Sometimes, despite using the strategies we've discussed, it is still hard to get that sucker to pass. Decreased coordination can cause reflexive, unintentional tension of your pelvic floor muscles (known as *anismus*) and could be contributing to the problem. With anismus, your pelvic floor muscles tighten, restricting the rectal opening, despite trying to relax. If this is the case, you'll want to consider seeing a pelvic floor physical therapist for a hands-on approach to improve your coordination.

Training for a Schedule

Like your bladder, your bowels are trainable too. Pick the most convenient time of the day and allow yourself ten minutes to sit on the toilet to try to stimulate a bowel movement. I know, I know, you don't possibly have ten minutes to try to sit to poop! Trust me, though; while you are using this time to train your bowels, you can also use these ten minutes to relax and meditate, and when you do have a bowel movement, positive endorphins get released! It's a win-win if you can budget this time into your day.

Part of the problem that goes hand in hand with constipation is that we are all so busy during the day, we don't take the time to listen to our bodies or give it the time it needs to function. When sitting on the toilet, be mindful to avoid straining; your goal is not to spend ten minutes actively pushing! Instead, try to completely relax and breathe easily to help stimulate your bowels to eliminate.

Here's a training sequence that works well:

1. Drink your water and/or warm liquid in the morning with breakfast.
2. Lie down to complete a three- to five-minute colon massage.
3. Sit on the toilet for ten minutes before you leave for work or before you start your activities for the day. Relax and breathe easily while sitting to help your body stimulate your bowels. Don't strain!

This will take you fifteen extra minutes at most, and if you can poop and spend your day not feeling constipated, I'd say those extra fifteen minutes are well worth it.

DIARRHEA

Loose stool, which appears as Type 6 or 7 on the Bristol Stool Chart, can be just as bothersome as constipation. When your poop is loose, it is harder for your external anal sphincter muscle to hold back the contents after your sampling reflex tells you that it's liquid coming down the tube. This, as you may imagine, can subject you to fecal incontinence (leaking stool).

If you struggle with loose stool, try the following strategies:

1. *Increase your soluble fiber:* With diarrhea, you want to increase soluble fiber to help bulk up your stool so it's more solid. Refer to Table 7 for sources of soluble fiber.

2. *Track your food:* Loose stool can stem from a dietary intolerance. If you can make a correlation to what you're eating and when you experience diarrhea, avoid eating that food. For example, if you can make a connection between loose stool and dairy, then you may be lactose intolerant. I'm speaking from experience here; before I discovered I was lactose intolerant, I had several close calls because of the quick onset of loose stool from eating dairy. Needless to say, this can ruin a fun trip for ice cream! If you are unable to figure out any connections through your own tracking, consult a healthcare provider such as a nutritionist or gastrointestinal doctor for further testing.

3. *Consult a pelvic floor physical therapist:* If you have a hard time maintaining continence of your bowels, feel bowel urgency, or have had "close calls" with your bowels, it may be due to coordination, reflex, strength, or tension issues within your pelvic floor. A thorough exam and pelvic floor muscle assessment can help determine the course of treatment you need. Don't accept this as a normal part of aging; it can be helped!

4. *Understand your emotions:* Have you even received upsetting news and felt instant knots in your stomach? There is a strong link between our emotions and our gut. If you begin to notice that you experience diarrhea during times of stress or adversity, you may benefit from counseling to help with your emotional health. If you fall into this category, recognize that there is absolutely no shame here! Think about how many of us would benefit from a counselor to help coach us through the ups and downs of life. In my opinion, we all would.

Table 7: Sources of Soluble Fiber to Bulk Stool

> *Carbohydrates:* Corn cereals, corn tortillas, oatmeal, pasta, quinoa, rice, rice cereals
>
> *Fruit:* mangos, bananas, avocados
>
> *Nuts:* chestnuts
>
> *Vegetables:* mushrooms, pumpkin, parsnips, beets, squash, sweet potatoes, rutabagas, carrots, yams, potatoes

IRRITABLE BOWEL SYNDROME (IBS)

As previously mentioned in the constipation section, there is an objective measure to help determine if you have IBS. For review, it includes recurrent abdominal pain more than one day per week in the last three months and two or more of the following criteria: a bowel movement that either increases or decreases pain; a change in bowel movement frequency; a change in stool type.

With IBS, there are three types of issues: constipation dominant, diarrhea dominant, or mixed. Regardless of the type, IBS presents in a painful, episodic, chronic nature. Emotions, such as stress, can especially impact the pain and bloating symptoms associated with IBS.

Due to the fluctuating presentation of IBS, dietary and supplement recommendations vary drastically. If you struggle with IBS, consult a gastrointestinal doctor for guidance on supplement and medication management, a nutritionist for personal diet recommendations, and of course a pelvic floor physical therapist to help ensure that your muscles are functioning optimally and that your toileting habits are superb.

FECAL INCONTINENCE

Just like you may experience urinary incontinence (bladder leaking), you can also experience fecal incontinence, which is also known as bowel leaking. Just like bladder leakage, bowel leakage is not normal and should not be accepted as a normal part of aging—ever. When I ask women if they have issues with leaking of their bowels, I always get one of two responses.

Some women say, "No, and thank God I don't have that problem. I didn't know that could happen." Other women drop their heads, embarrassed, and softly say, "Yes, I have that problem." From my experience, bowel leakage is not as well known or talked about as bladder leakage is, but it is still just as annoying and embarrassing, perhaps even more so.

You may recall from chapter 4, "Bladder Health," that urinary incontinence can present itself whether you have weak or tight pelvic floor muscles. Well, the same is true with fecal incontinence. If your pelvic floor muscles are already tight, then they will not be able to squeeze to engage any further when you are trying to hold back stool, which means Kegels will only make the problem worse. If your pelvic floor muscles are weak, then they will lack the strength to squeeze to engage to close the rectal opening, which means that Kegels can help. Consequently, it is imperative to know which route you need—lengthening or strengthening—both of which are thoroughly covered in chapter 7, "To Lengthen or Strengthen." Let's now take a closer look at just how fecal incontinence can be classified:

1. *Urge fecal incontinence:* This occurs when you have a really strong urge to go and cannot hold it, just like urge urinary incontinence. When your colon sends a sample and your body identifies that you have solid stool or liquid stool wanting to pass, normally your pelvic floor muscles will squeeze to engage, holding back the stool until you've reached the toilet. However, in this case the urge to go is so strong, you can't hold it back. Remember, this can occur because your muscles are already in a tense position and cannot squeeze any further or because they are too weak to squeeze. You may experience this issue with either stool that is loose or stool that is formed, but it is most common with loose stool. If your fecal incontinent stool is loose, then you may have an underlying dietary intolerance or a lack of soluble fiber. (See the earlier discussion of these problems.) If your fecal incontinent stool is formed, then the cause is likely more to be an issue with your pelvic floor muscles' inability to close off the anal opening until you've reached the toilet.

2. *Passive fecal incontinence:* This occurs when you leak stool but are not aware of doing so (it's passive). This can be really challenging to deal with because you never know when it's going to strike. Like urge fecal incontinence, this usually happens when stool is loose, which again can be caused from dietary intolerances or lack of soluble fiber. Additionally, because you aren't aware of when this is happening, it's safe to say that your body is having a hard time sensing the sample coming down. Treating this successfully often requires sensory and coordination training from a pelvic floor physical therapist.

3. *Mixed fecal incontinence:* You guessed it: this occurs when you experience both urge and passive fecal incontinence. Usually one problem is worse than the other and began prior to the other. Regardless, it's important to address both.

4. *Overflow fecal incontinence:* This occurs when you are incontinent of loose stool that overflows and seeps around compacted, stuck stool. This can be common with chronic constipation as your body tries to eliminate the stool matter that is trapped behind the stuck part. This can be classified as either urge or passive fecal incontinence. You'll know you fall into this category if you experience fecal incontinence with constipation.

Regardless of which type of fecal incontinence you may be experiencing, pelvic floor physical therapy can help! Rest assured that there is no need to feel embarrassed about this when talking to your healthcare providers; we are here to help.

HEMORRHOIDS

The dreaded hemorrhoid. We've all heard of it, but what exactly is it, and how does it even happen? A hemorrhoid is a swollen vein in the rectal or anal area that can develop for many reasons.

Hemorrhoids develop either internally or externally. An internal rectal hemorrhoid usually flies under the radar unseen, but don't be fooled, it can still cause discomfort when having a bowel movement, and if it is swollen enough, it will protrude through the anal opening. An external anal hemorrhoid is very much visible and can cause itching, pain, swelling, and bleeding around the anal opening.

Hemorrhoids can be triggered by anything that places extra pressure on the rectal and anal opening, causing the veins to stretch and swell. For example, holding back your poop, straining to poop, sitting for long periods of time (more than twenty minutes) on the toilet, chronic constipation or diarrhea, incontinence, obesity, pregnancy, heavy lifting with the Valsalva maneuver, and a low-fiber diet can all contribute.

Usually, hemorrhoids will calm down with simple home remedies. These include taking warm baths, using a hot compress, applying topical hemorrhoid creams, and—most important—avoiding the contributing factors mentioned above. If you have a hemorrhoid that is not going away on its own, consult your healthcare provider for further treatment options.

CHAPTER SIX

Pelvic Pain

"To be heard, believed,
and validated is powerful.
To have a plan for healing
is life-changing."

—Dr. Megan Rorabeck, DPT, WCS

Pelvic pain did not become a true clinical diagnosis until 2013.[19] Prior to this time it was labeled a psychiatric disorder. Thankfully, pelvic pain has become a more recognized issue with improvement in appropriate referrals and treatments.

I have treated numerous patients with pelvic pain. Several of them saw multiple healthcare providers prior to finding their way to pelvic floor physical therapy—and they were all grateful for the relief it finally gave them.

Sad but true, oftentimes patients are not taken seriously when they mention pelvic pain to their healthcare provider. It takes courage for patients to raise this issue, so any response that shrugs off the problem and offers no solution is heartbreaking. I've heard comments from patients such as these:

"My doctor told me it's normal because I'm getting older and I've had kids."

"My doctor told me this is just part of the aging process; it's normal."

"I've been labeled a drug seeker because of my emergency department visits for the pain."

"I was told to just drink some wine when it hurts."

If your jaw is on the floor right now, mine was too when I heard these responses. I realize that medical providers have limited time with patients, are often overbooked, and frequently have had limited education and training on pelvic pain diagnoses, but it is still absolutely unacceptable for them to give these types of responses. In many cases, you will have to be your own best advocate to find and receive the care you need and deserve. After reading this chapter, I hope you gain just that.

THE BENEFITS OF COLLABORATION

As you've probably gathered, there are many factors to consider with pelvic pain. Pelvic pain can be driven from the digestive, gastrointestinal, urological, reproductive, nervous, or musculoskeletal system, or it can be psychogenic in nature. It can be due to one system, a combination of a few of them, or all systems. No single provider is fully capable of providing comprehensive treatment within all systems, and that is why a collaborative approach for diagnosis and treatment is absolutely necessary.

A gynecologist can check for infections and sexually transmitted diseases. A urologist can do a bladder scope to look at the inner lining of your bladder. A nutritionist and gastroenterologist can identify dietary intolerances. A mental health counselor can help you work through traumas or mood instabilities related to your well-being. A physical therapist can address the nervous system and musculoskeletal system to identify and treat bony malalignments, trigger points within muscles, and oversensitive nerves—just to name a few treatment options. You are a *whole* person, and to properly address your needs as a whole, it usually takes a team. For this reason, it's essential that you advocate for yourself and what you need. It may take some searching, but it is definitely in your best interest to find healthcare providers who advocate for you, who are willing to be on your team, and who truly want to make a difference for you in your life. I also understand that this process can be overwhelming, time-consuming, and expensive. In my opinion, seeking help from a pelvic floor physical therapist is a great place to start. As physical therapists, part of our job is to help you determine which providers you may also need to see and to explain to you why you'd need to see them. We can help you figure out next best steps so you can coordinate and plan of your care without feeling too overwhelmed.

DIAGNOSES

To go over every pelvic pain diagnosis in detail is beyond the scope of this book; there are entire books written on single diagnoses! I do, however, want to provide a brief description of common diagnoses to help you better understand and communicate this information to your healthcare provider. Here they are.

Coccygodynia

The word *coccygodynia* means "tailbone pain." Your tailbone joins the sacrum, forming a joint that normally moves five to twenty-five degrees. As you now know, the tailbone serves as an attachment point for several of the deep, third-layer pelvic floor muscles. Your tailbone has to move every time your spine moves. Tailbone pain can be present for a variety of reasons, including (but not limited to) the following:

- Tight or weak pelvic floor muscles
- Tight or weak glute (or butt cheek) muscles
- Poor posture, especially when sitting
- A too mobile or too stiff tailbone
- Constipation

Dysmenorrhea

Dysmenorrhea is defined as painful periods. It is another common misconception that painful periods are normal. Yes, your uterus is shedding its lining so mild cramps make sense, but debilitating pain that leaves you curled up in the fetal position, missing work, or taking time off school is not normal.

Dyspareunia

Dyspareunia is pelvic pain or discomfort associated with attempted vaginal penetration (e.g., with intercourse or tampon insertion). Dyspareunia has many defining subcategories:

- *Superficial or deep:* Pain can be experienced as superficial pain at the vaginal opening with initial vaginal penetration, deep pain with deep vaginal penetration, or both.
- *Generalized or situational:* Pain can be generalized, where it is present with all encounters of vaginal penetration. Pain can be situational, where it is only present in certain situations or with certain partners.
- *Primary or secondary:* The onset of pain can be primary, since the first time of attempted vaginal penetration (e.g., with intercourse or tampon insertion), or secondary, where onset of pain occurs after a previously pain-free period of vaginal penetration.

No matter which subcategory your pain falls into, the underlying cause of dyspareunia still needs to be addressed. The underlying cause can stem from a number of diagnoses, such as an infection, vaginismus, endometriosis, inadequate lubrication, vulvar vestibulitis syndrome, etc. It is important to identify the underlying cause of dyspareunia to determine the best course of treatment. Your gynecologist and pelvic floor physical therapist will help you with this.

Endometriosis

Endometriosis occurs when endometrial tissue, which normally lines the inside of your uterus, grows outside of your uterus. Pain usually occurs because this endometrial tissue swells and bleeds during menses but cannot easily leave your body during your period because it's not actually inside your uterus. The pain is cyclical and chronic. Endometrial tissue can grow near the ovaries, fallopian tubes, bladder, and bowel, contributing to adhesions and more pain.

Interstitial Cystitis (IC) and Overactive Bladder (OAB)

Interstitial cystitis (IC), which is also referred to as painful bladder syndrome, is thought to occur when foods and fluids more easily irritate the bladder lining, causing sensitivity and inflammation. Ulcerations may or may not be present in the bladder. Overactive bladder (OAB) can sometimes be confused with IC. The key differences include the following:

IC = pain with bladder filling, urinating frequently to relieve pain, strong urges

OAB = urinating frequently to avoid leakage, strong urges

Lichens Sclerosus

Lichens sclerosus mostly affects postmenopausal women, and its cause is unknown. It is a condition causing white, thinned tissue patches in the vulva. Symptoms typically include itching, pain, discomfort, and easily torn tissues and bleeding, which results in pain during intercourse. If you experience these symptoms and notice white patches surrounding your vaginal opening (all the more reason to grab a mirror and look down there!), consult your doctor, who may prescribe a topical cream/ointment as well as pelvic floor physical therapy to address the likely tight surrounding pelvic floor muscles.

Pelvic Congestion Syndrome (PCS)

Pelvic congestion syndrome (PCS) is analogous to having varicose veins in your pelvis. With PCS, the veins within your pelvis have a decreased ability to return blood to your heart (the normal role of veins). Thus, blood pools in the veins, causing further swelling, and thus pain. It is not fully understood what causes PCS, but it is thought that estrogen, which has a "relaxing" effect on veins, especially during pregnancy, may contribute.

Pelvic Inflammatory Disease (PID)

Pelvic inflammatory disease (PID) is an infection of the reproductive organs caused by sexually transmitted diseases. Unlike other pelvic pain diagnoses, with PID you may not experience pain immediately; it can go undetected. Signs and symptoms to be mindful of include abdominal pain, fever, odorous discharge, pain or bleeding with intercourse, bleeding between periods, and UTI-like symptoms.

Proctalgia Fugax

Proctalgia fugax is a fancy way of saying sharp, fleeting rectal pain. The underlying cause must still be addressed and determined with the help of your healthcare providers. Usually, there will be thickening and spasming of the internal anal sphincter muscle, a second-layer pelvic floor muscle. This means there is a component of tight pelvic floor muscles and potential nerve irritation, which a pelvic floor physical therapist can address.

Pudendal neuralgia

Pudendal neuralgia is irritation of the pudendal nerve. From chapter 1, "The Pelvic Girdle," you know this nerve takes quite a long, complicated path from the back of the sacrum to the pelvic floor muscles, dividing into three branches. (Refer back to that chapter for the exact details!) With pudendal neuralgia, the pudendal nerve can become irritated anywhere along its path. You may experience itching, burning, tingling, and/or muscle spasms. Your bowel and bladder function may also be affected. Usually, pain will be aggravated with tight clothing and sitting—anything that further compresses the nerve. Sometimes, sitting on a toilet seat is not as provocative because there is no pressure placed on the pelvic floor area itself.

Vaginismus

Vaginismus is a spasming or a reflexive contraction of the pelvic floor muscles upon attempted vaginal penetration, preventing penetration. Similar to dyspareunia, vaginismus has defining subcategories:

Primary: You have never been able to tolerate vaginal penetration.

Secondary: The vaginismus developed after a pain-free period of time.

Again, your healthcare providers must determine the underlying cause of vaginismus. Both primary and secondary vaginismus are thought to be due to a negative experience such as trauma or abuse. In that case, counseling would be a recommended treatment in addition to pelvic floor physical therapy to address the tightness and pain within the pelvic floor muscles.

Vulvodynia

Vulvodynia is defined as a burning, stinging, or raw feeling within the vaginal opening that can be associated with vaginismus and dyspareunia; sometimes the vaginal opening may look red and irritated. The underlying cause of vulvodynia will need to be addressed by your healthcare provider. Abuse and trauma, vaginal infections, and postmenopausal status are some factors that may contribute to vulvodynia.

GETTING HELP

Now that you have information about a few possible diagnoses for pelvic pain, how can you work with healthcare professionals to establish a plan for healing? As I've mentioned, treating pelvic pain is truly a multidisciplinary approach, with collaboration between all providers. For example, this may include a primary care provider (PCP), gynecologist, urologist, counselor, nutritionist, and pelvic floor physical therapist.

As you probably noticed, several of the pain diagnoses can overlap. Someone with endometriosis may also experience deep dyspareunia. To identify the true underlying cause of your pain, it is important that you have your medical provider perform a thorough assessment. For example, pelvic inflammatory disease can be caused by a sexually transmitted disease like gonorrhea. If that is the case, the disease should be treated first by a PCP or gynecologist prior to or in conjunction with pelvic floor physical therapy. In some US states, you do not need a referral from a medical doctor to attend physical therapy. It is then the physical therapist's job to assess the need for a referral to other providers for additional medical testing and collaboration. In other states, you will need a doctor to refer you. In either case, let's look at what may happen once you make the appointment with the pelvic floor physical therapist.

In our example, let's say that you arrive for your first appointment for pelvic floor physical therapy with a referral from your gynecologist. Now what? You will first be asked to fill out intake paperwork. This paperwork is used to help track objective progress, and if you are being treated through insurance, it helps authorize coverage for care. After the paperwork is finished, we get down to business! Your pelvic floor physical therapist will first simply talk with you to better understand what is going on. This will include asking you questions about your past medical history, your bladder and bowel health, the details surrounding your pain, and any other relevant issues. Usually, in the presence of pelvic pain, there will also be bladder and/or bowel issues because of the close relationship of everything between the hips.

Next, as part of the objective examination, if you agree and if you find it tolerable, your physical therapist will perform an internal pelvic floor muscle assessment with one gloved finger vaginally or rectally. Sometimes, this is done at the second visit if you prefer to wait. This postponement is okay because the physical therapist can still use the first visit to assess (at a minimum) your spine, belly, and hips.

Believe it or not, physical therapists can actually assess all of your pelvic floor muscles via the vaginal canal and rectal canal. However, if you can't tolerate an internal muscle assessment due to pain or personal preference, the therapist will do an external assessment as the next best alternative.

After the pelvic floor muscle assessment, your treatment options will depend on the findings. For instance, you might need to lengthen or strengthen your pelvic floor muscles. In the next chapter, I'll help you understand what your treatment options might look like.

AN ALIGNMENT EXERCISE THAT BENEFITS ALL WOMEN

Before we move on, I'd like to share an exercise that everyone can benefit from because it helps ensure that your pelvic girdle is properly aligned, which allows your pelvic floor muscles to do their job of contracting, relaxing, opening, and supporting more effectively. Without this correction, if your pelvic girdle is rotated, then the pelvic floor muscles follow suit—being pulled and tensed—which can contribute to pelvic floor dysfunction.

What causes the pelvic girdle to rotate out of alignment? You may recall that the pelvic girdle has the pubic symphysis joint in the front and sacroiliac joints in the back. At these locations, your pelvis can shift ever so slightly, particularly when you bend, lift, carry, exercise, or use poor posture and body mechanics during the day. To avoid unwarranted panic, I want to make clear that it is not necessarily a bad thing if your pelvis isn't exactly aligned. However, if you experience pelvic symptoms—including bladder issues, bowel issues, and/or pain—it can be beneficial to address this.

Muscles have memory, and if your pelvis is rotated out of alignment, your muscles will remember this unideal position. To combat this problem, you must reestablish a neutral, properly aligned position for your body to remember, which is done by correcting your pelvis often and using good pelvic posture. In fact, you'll want to correct your pelvis two or three times per day, especially after high-level activity. The correction, which is illustrated in figure 35, goes as follows:

1. Lie on your back on the floor or on your bed, with your knees bent and your feet flat on the floor. Lift your butt up off the floor and then place it back down. Just a quick up and down. This helps ensure your pelvis is in a neutral position where your low back is not excessively arched or pressed flat against the floor. There should be a small, natural curve of your low back against the floor.

2. Lift one leg up toward you, so your upper thigh forms a ninety-degree angle with your hip and your knee is bent in a relaxed position. Reach behind the crook of your knee with both hands, interlacing your fingers. Your elbows will be relatively straight and your shoulders should be relaxed.

3. Push your leg into your hands for two deep breaths. Your hands will block the motion of the push so your upper thigh remains at a ninety-degree angle with your hip. After pushing your leg into your hands, place your leg back down in the starting position where your knees are bent and feet flat on the floor.

4. Repeat the exercise with the other leg.

5. Perform three rounds of pushing each leg into your hands, alternating between each leg.

That's it! It is very easy, and it will feel like you're doing almost nothing at all.

Figure 35: Pelvic Correction Exercise

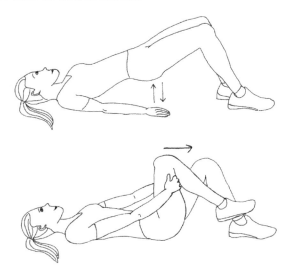

So, how exactly does this work? This is a technique that uses an isometric contraction, which means there is muscle activation in the absence of a body part moving. Therefore, the muscle force generated helps to properly align the pelvic girdle.

As an attestation to how much this simple exercise can help, I've had women present with a longstanding history of pelvic pain and/or back pain. At our initial appointment, we usually have so much medical history to cover, I have enough time only to teach them this correction. Even so, *with just this correction,* most of them return feeling the best they have felt since their symptoms began.

I also do this correction daily in my own life. Many years ago, I hurt the left side of my low back when my sister was teaching me how to twerk. Yes, you read that right. For those who don't know, twerking is a dance move where you squat and shake your booty really fast. I've had on-and-off back pain with left-sided pelvic floor spasms ever since. However, this pelvic correction helps me manage my pain—even if my dance moves are still on hold!

CHAPTER SEVEN

To Lengthen or Strengthen

"The willow is my favorite tree.
I grew up near one. It's the most flexible tree
in nature and nothing can break it—no wind,
no elements, it can bend and withstand anything."

—Pink

PERHAPS ALONG YOUR ROAD to treatment you've been advised to "try doing Kegels." This catch-phrase answer is often provided to women who are seeking advice for issues between their hips. I hate to sound like a Negative Nancy here, but it's usually never that simple. As you can see from the information in the previous chapters, you must address your habits and behaviors around your bladder and bowels. Kegels alone will not change these habits, and therefore they usually will not provide any relief when done alone. No matter what your age or your obstetrics history, the information in this section is applicable.

In this chapter, I'll share more tools you can add to your comprehensive treatment plan. We will review key information about tight and weak pelvic floor muscles, and I'll explain the treatment options that can help you lengthen or strengthen your pelvic floor to achieve optimal pelvic health. Please keep in mind that my goal here is to help you better understand what could be going on with your pelvic floor and what your treatment options are so you can communicate this information with your doctor or physical therapist for further guidance. You will still want a professional diagnosis—don't try to diagnose yourself! You should always have a qualified healthcare provider such as your gynecologist or your pelvic floor physical therapist—not your friends, not Google—identify if you have tight muscles that need to be lengthened or weak muscles that need to be strengthened. For instance, your gynecologist or pelvic floor physical therapist can check your muscles by doing a vaginal or rectal exam and address the other questions or concerns you have with issues between your hips.

Generally, the presence or absence of pain can provide insight into how your muscles present: tight or weak. When your pelvic floor muscles are stuck tight, it's painful. The following symptoms of pelvic or abdominal pain often indicate that your muscles are tight and you must lengthen them:

- Pain with intercourse or with tampon use
- Pain with gynecological exams
- Abdominal, low back, hip, sit bone, or back-of-the-thigh pain
- Inability to tolerate tight clothing
- Feelings of burning or rawness in or around your vagina
- Feeling like you are clenching your pelvic floor or butt muscles

You may also wish to review the diagnosis section of chapter 6.

As recommended in chapter 3, "Between the Hips Sexy Self-Care," you should take a look at your perineum monthly. This can also cue you in on any pelvic floor tension. When the pelvic floor muscles are tight, they restrict blood flow to this area, resulting in a darker than normal color. If your labia (the outer lips) look darker in color than normal, dark red or purple, it may indicate a decreased sump-pump function of the pelvic floor muscles (see chapter 1, "The Pelvic Girdle"). However, even if your perineum is not darker in color, you can still have tension and pain within your pelvic floor muscles.

In contrast, you probably have weak (versus tight and painful) pelvic floor muscles if your situation reflects the following:

- You do not experience pain—meaning you never, and I really mean never, have pain with the situations highlighted in the previous list.
- You do not feel that you clench or hold tight your core, butt cheek, or pelvic floor muscles.

- You feel your pelvic floor is weak.
- You have not noticed a darkening color of your tissues.

This is not to say that women with weak pelvic floor muscles cannot experience pelvic floor muscle pain, but it is less likely.

Since bladder and bowel issues such as leakage can occur with both tight and weak pelvic floor muscles, they cannot be the sole factor to determine if your muscles are tight or weak. Again, I would recommend having an actual pelvic floor muscle assessment by your gynecologist or pelvic floor physical therapist to exactly determine where you are. Once you have a diagnosis, you can consider your treatment options, which we'll explore next.

TIGHT PELVIC FLOOR MUSCLES

Imagine walking around with your shoulders hiked up to your ears all day . . . OUCH! This analogy explains what it is like to have tight pelvic floor muscles. Oftentimes, it is challenging for patients to even feel what is going on down there! Consequently, you may find it hard to try to relax your muscles because you may not even be able to feel the tension in the first place. Here are more cues to help you identify if you may be clenching your pelvic floor:

The mouth cue: If you are clenching your jaw or grinding your teeth, you are more prone to be clenching your pelvic floor, since they serve as the two openings of the body. If you feel tension in your jaw, or even in your neck, you may be clenching your pelvic floor.

The bum cue: The glutes, or butt cheek muscles, sit right next door to your pelvic floor. If you feel clenching or tension within your bum, you may be tensing your pelvic floor. Because these muscles are essentially neighbors, when one contracts, the other may do so as well.

The stress ball cue: We've all been there, trying to divide our attention between ten different tasks, running late, using a white-knuckle-grip on the steering wheel, or hunching over a computer, vigorously working away and hardly remembering to breathe. In these situations, you are likely holding your body, and thus your pelvic floor, tense.

I'm sure at some point we've all been in a situation where we clench our jaw, experience tension in our neck, or feel stressed. However, if you find yourself in any or all of these situations—mouth clenching, bum clenching, or stress balling—take your attention to your pelvic floor and ask yourself if you feel like you're clenching there too. This step can help improve your awareness of your pelvic floor. Even if you can't determine with confidence whether your pelvic floor is clenching or not, relaxation strategies such as deep breathing, meditating, and gentle exercise like walking or yoga can help. (I know what you're thinking: you're stressed or running late and I'm asking you to s l o w d o w n. Yes, trust me, you will feel better after!) The next section explores some great options specifically to help stretch and relax your pelvic floor if it is tight.

Breathing

A simple way to stretch your pelvic floor and help you relax is deep breathing. Instead of adopting a short, upper-chest breathing pattern, you will want to try a deep, belly-breathing pattern like what is commonly practiced in yoga. I want to actually teach you how to do this correctly, because it will help relax your pelvic floor *and* your mind!

The easiest way to learn is to begin by lying on your back with one hand on your belly and one on your chest. The goal is to have your belly hand move more than your chest hand, indicating that you are breathing deep into your belly. Keep in mind the close relationship between the core muscles and pelvic floor muscles—what one area does, the other area does! When you inhale, your diaphragm pulls down, your belly rises up so that your abdominal muscles lengthen to stretch, and your pelvic floor muscles lengthen to stretch. (You may not feel anything in your pelvic floor yet, but that's okay.) This type of belly breathing is not a vigorous or gasping inhale. Focus on a natural exchange of air, simply pulling your breath deep. Figure 36 illustrates how the core and pelvic floor muscles both lengthen to stretch when you inhale.

Figure 36: Belly Breathing to Stretch Your Pelvic Floor

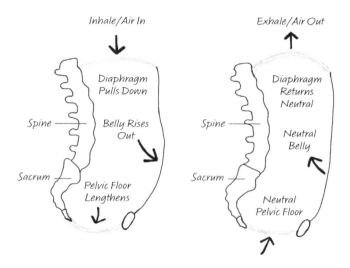

Once you feel you've got the hang of it lying down, try this breathing strategy as you are sitting in a chair. With this approach, you may be able to better feel your pelvic floor lengthen. Remember, your pelvic floor sits in the area between your sit bones, which are literally the bones you sit on, and it's the area of your "lady parts." You should feel this area lengthen, swell, and stretch out into the chair surface when you inhale.

Next, try this exercise while you are standing. You can use this breathing strategy anytime, anywhere, anyplace. It's a tool you'll always have in your toolbox.

As an additional bonus, you can use this breathing strategy as a form of meditative work by relaxing comfortably flat on your back or in seated position and solely focusing on your breathing for up to ten minutes. If you do this once a day for ten minutes, you should find that overall you feel more calm and relaxed!

Dilators and Pelvic Floor Muscle Wands

Another treatment option to directly stretch tight pelvic floor muscles through the vaginal and/or rectal opening is to use a dilator or a wand. Figure 37 shows examples of each.

This is another situation where you should not rush in to diagnose yourself. Instead, it is best to consult a pelvic floor physical therapist to help determine if you would need a wand or a dilator and to guide you through the techniques on how to use them to directly release your pelvic floor muscles. Dilators and wands can be ordered online; they may also be available directly from your physical therapist's office. Here's a quick explanation on how dilators and wands work.

Dilators primarily stretch the first and second layers of the pelvic floor muscles. They are made of plastic or silicone and come in a variety of circumferential sizes and lengths. A pelvic floor physical therapist will help you determine which size to start with. When using a dilator, you'll want to be relaxed. If you are using the dilator vaginally, lying on your back works best, and if you are using it rectally, lying on your side can be more comfortable. Be sure to apply lubricant to decrease friction and improve comfort.

Figure 37: Dilators and Wands

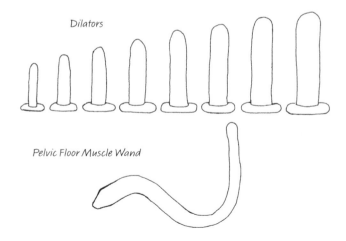

Dilators

Pelvic Floor Muscle Wand

Insert the dilator as far as your body will tolerate it comfortably. Every woman's vaginal length is different, but don't be afraid of inserting the dilator too far. You will either hit a point where it is uncomfortable or you will nudge your cervix. In either case, if it is uncomfortable, simply back it out a bit to a point where it is comfortable. Once you have the dilator inserted to a tolerable length, practice breathing, meditating, or any relaxation strategy.

Wands are "S" shaped and primarily stretch the deepest, third layer of your pelvic floor muscles. The third layer sits like a hammock slinging from your pubic bone to your tailbone, and a wand can better stretch these hammock-like muscles than a dilator can. Again, being sure to use lubricant, insert the wand to the level of the third layer, about one full pointer-finger-length in, and sweep it across the tight muscles to gently stretch them via light pressure.

Pelvic floor muscle dilators and wands are usually used for up to ten minutes, once a day. Ten minutes is ample—in this case, longer isn't better. The time of day is completely up to you, but consistency is key here. Aim to stretch for a short period of time (e.g., ten minutes) every day versus a longer period of time (e.g., thirty minutes) only a few times a week. You can also use your dilator or wand to pre-stretch your pelvic floor muscles, again for up to ten minutes, prior to having penetrative intercourse to help decrease pain. Using them prior to intercourse may take some of the spontaneity away, but it can lead to a more comfortable experience.

Postponing Kegels

As I'm sure you now realize, there is so much more to treating the pelvic floor than just doing Kegels! In fact, when the pelvic floor muscles are already tight and tense, which is often the case with pelvic pain —then you *should not do Kegels!* In this case, it's important to avoid further tensing of these muscles. Once your muscles have lengthened, *then* you will want to address strengthening by doing Kegels. Your physical therapist can help you determine when you are ready to begin Kegels.

Stretching

Another strategy to help decrease tightness within your pelvic floor is stretching. Your pelvic floor muscles attach to the pelvic girdle, as do several hip and spine muscles. If you add in the breathing strategy mentioned earlier, you get a two-for-one stretch! Table 8 includes some common stretches to help relax your pelvic floor. You'll want to hold each stretch for sixty seconds and perform them two times a day.

Table 8: Stretches to Decrease Pelvic Floor Tightness

STRETCH	AREA STRETCHED
Child's Pose Stretch (figure 38)	Mid-low back and glutes (butt cheeks)
Hamstring Stretch (figure 39)	Back of your thigh
Psoas Stretch (figure 40)	Front of your hip and side of your trunk on the down-knee side
Butterfly Stretch (figure 41)	Groin

The stretches are shown in more detail in figures 38, 39, 40, and 41. (The psoas stretch also appeared as figure 30.) Here are the written instructions.

Child's pose stretch (figure 38): Start by kneeling with your knees wide and feet touching. Sit back on your heels and stretch your arms out in front of you on the ground.

Figure 38: Child's Pose Stretch

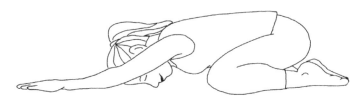

Hamstring stretch (figure 39): Sit at the edge of a chair with one leg out straight in front of you so your heel is down and your knee is straight. Lean forward as far as you feel comfortable, bending at your waist. Repeat on the other side.

Figure 39: Hamstring Stretch

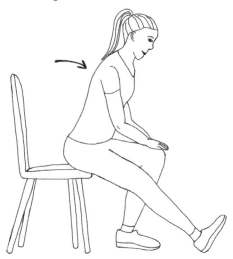

Psoas stretch (figure 40): Kneel so your right knee is on a pillow and your left foot is planted in front of you. Keep your hips pointing straight ahead and your chest tall and straight. Reach your right arm overhead, feeling a stretch through the front of your right hip and into the right side of your trunk. Repeat on the other side, using your left knee and arm. You will feel the second stretch on your left hip and into the left side of your trunk.

Figure 40: Psoas Stretch

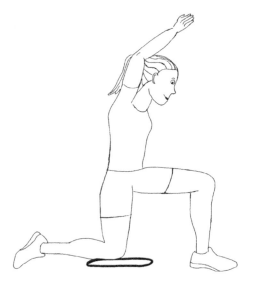

Butterfly stretch (figure 41): Sit upright against a wall. Then bend your knees so the soles of your feet are together and as close to you as comfortable. If needed, use a pillow between each knee and the floor for added support.

Figure 41: Butterfly Stretch

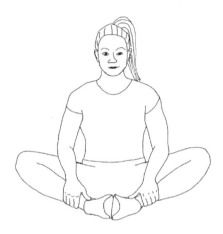

Soft Tissue Mobilization (STM)

All of the strategies thus far have described options you can do independently to help relax and stretch your pelvic floor muscles if they are tight. Soft tissue mobilization (STM), which is done by a pelvic floor physical therapist, is another way to stretch your pelvic floor to directly release tense and tight tissue, including tight pelvic floor muscles, pelvic ligaments, and the tissue around nerves. STM can be done vaginally, rectally, or externally over your hips, spine, sacrum, abdomen, and thighs. It specifically targets, releases, and stretches the tense tissue—all the more reason to consult a pelvic floor physical therapist!

WEAK PELVIC FLOOR MUSCLES

Before we dive into this discussion, try to confirm if your muscles are truly weak. Believe it or not, pelvic muscles that feel weak may actually be muscles that are stuck tight (see the previous section). To understand how this might be the case, let's go back to the analogy of having your shoulders hiked to your ears and how that situation can be similar to having tight pelvic floor muscles. In this case, imagine your shoulders are hiked all the way up to your ears, but you aren't *aware* of your shoulders being in this position. Then, if someone asks you to lift your shoulders to your ears, you can't do it—not because of a weakness, but because your shoulders are already there! However, you may erroneously perceive this as a weakness.

This is the same way your pelvic floor works. If you're already holding your pelvic floor muscles tight but are not aware of it, then when you try to squeeze your pelvic floor (say, to do a Kegel), you feel minimal to no movement, which you perceive as weakness. For the rest of this section, we will assume that your pelvic floor is truly weak and explore what kinds of treatment may help.

How to Kegel

It is important to know how to properly Kegel and strengthen your pelvic floor muscles. I have only worked with a handful of people who Kegel correctly without needing cuing or help. There are a lot of ways your body will cheat to try to make it easier.

If you recall from the very first chapter, "The Pelvic Girdle," you learned that the transverse abdominis muscle, which is the deep corset-like core muscle, and your pelvic floor muscles are best friends. They help and support each other with everything, and you bet that continues when you are doing Kegels too! When you are doing a Kegel correctly, your pelvic floor muscles and the deep core muscle squeeze to engage—nothing more. In other words, you want to *avoid* adding any of the following movements, which are also called *compensations*:

- Holding your breath
- Sucking in your stomach
- Clenching your bum (glutes or butt cheek muscles)
- Squeezing your inner thigh muscles

- Arching or flattening your back
- Bearing down, which is also known as pushing (discussed shortly!)

When you are doing a Kegel, try using these cues to help isolate your core and your pelvic floor:

- *Core:* Using just your muscles, squeeze to pull your belly button up under your rib cage.
- *Core:* Pull your belly button toward your spine by squeezing to engage your core. Do not suck in your abdomen, but rather squeeze it.
- *Pelvic floor:* Squeeze like you're trying to hold back urine or gas.
- *Pelvic floor:* Imagine trying to squeeze your muscles tight around a tampon in your vagina.
- *Pelvic floor:* Imagine that your vagina has a straw to a very thick milkshake; use your pelvic floor muscles only to suck up the milkshake.

Now that you know which compensations you should avoid and which cues can help you isolate your core and pelvic floor, let's walk through the sequence of how it all goes together.

When you are first starting to practice Kegels, use your breathing, particularly the exhale, to help. This approach is effective because as you exhale, your diaphragm, belly, and pelvic floor all return to a resting position (after they lengthened for the inhale), which makes the Kegel easier to do. Try this:

1. Lie on your back and inhale so your belly rises up toward the ceiling.
2. Exhale and notice how your belly falls.
3. On the next exhale, squeeze to engage your pelvic floor muscles and your core muscles, thinking about one of the cues above. Once you've initiated the Kegel on the exhale, you must continue to breathe while you maintain the Kegel; try counting out loud.
4. Release the Kegel, ensuring complete pelvic floor muscle relaxation by inhaling. Then, you may perform another Kegel.

This is a great time to grab a hand mirror to confirm that you are doing Kegels correctly. Watch carefully as you try a Kegel. You should see only the perineum moving *upward*. You should not see your butt cheeks moving. Earlier I mentioned that a common compensation is bearing down, also known as pushing. Make sure you are not actually pushing when you should be squeezing.

I also want to stress this important point: don't get frustrated if your Kegel doesn't feel right or look right. Doing a Kegel correctly can be more challenging than it sounds. Give yourself time to practice this, and be patient with yourself. As always, you can consult with a pelvic floor physical therapist to ensure that you're doing it correctly.

Kegel Positions

Certain positions make it easier to perform a Kegel due to gravity, which we know pulls everything down! As we've just discussed, at first you should practice when you are lying on your back. This is the easiest position because when you squeeze, you do not have to lift directly against gravity.

Once you feel you've got the hang of doing a Kegel correctly lying down, try it while you are sitting. Sitting is more challenging because now when you squeeze, you must squeeze against gravity. As you Kegel when you are sitting, you can feel your pelvic floor lifting up away from the seat's surface. If you squeeze and your whole body moves, then you've done too much and are recruiting helper muscles. You should be able to do a Kegel sitting in a chair in a room full of people and nobody will ever know! When you're stopped at a red light, Kegel. When there's a commercial on TV, Kegel. Sitting at work in a boring meeting? You guessed it: Kegel!

Standing is the hardest position of all because you're lifting against gravity, and you lose the cue of lifting up away from a seat. Being able to Kegel while standing is absolutely necessary because your pelvic floor needs to squeeze in order to get you to the bathroom leak-free when you have an urge to go. Be especially mindful of not clenching your butt cheek muscles when you practice Kegels while you are standing.

It is imperative to feel your pelvic floor muscles relax after you release the Kegel. If you are unable to feel your pelvic floor muscles relax, take a belly breath to ensure that these muscles are lengthening. (Remember, we discussed breathing earlier in the chapter.) If you do not relax your pelvic floor muscles after you Kegel, you run the risk of promoting tension and eventually pain. Let's use an elevator analogy to drive this point home. When your pelvic floor muscles are relaxed, imagine you're in an elevator on the ground floor. When you Kegel and squeeze to engage your pelvic floor, the elevator moves to the top floor. When you relax, you must let your pelvic floor (the elevator) return to its resting position (the ground floor). If you are struggling with this, please consult a pelvic floor physical therapist!

Two Kinds of Kegels

There are two kinds of Kegels in this world: sprints and marathons. As you may recall from the anatomy lesson at the start of the book, just like every muscle in your body, your pelvic floor muscles are made up of two kinds of muscle fibers—Type 1 (slow twitch/marathons) and Type 2 (fast twitch/sprints)—and we must address both fiber types. For example, you need your pelvic floor muscles to support your bladder while you are en route to the bathroom (a marathon), *and* you need your pelvic floor muscles to quickly squeeze when you sneeze, laugh, or lift (a sprint).

So how exactly do you train your pelvic floor muscles to be good sprinters and good marathoners? The answer: Kegel hold time. A longer Kegel hold time of five to ten seconds will address the marathon fibers, while a shorter Kegel hold time of two to four seconds will address the sprint fibers. The key rule still applies when you are trying to do a ten-second hold: you must feel *only* your pelvic floor and core squeezing to engage, nothing more.

To determine how long you can hold your Kegel, begin by lying on your back. Do a Kegel and count how many seconds you can maintain a good, strong squeeze. It is important to focus on the *quality* of your

Kegel. You will know it's time to stop because once you get tired, you will notice you are doing the following:

- Holding your breath
- Sucking in your stomach
- Using other muscles to help by clenching your glutes (butt cheek muscles) and your groin (inner thigh) muscles
- Experiencing leg trembles from fatigue
- Moving your spine so that it arches up or flattens down into the ground
- Losing the engagement you initially felt with your pelvic floor muscle squeeze (that is, you now feel the elevator dropping to the ground floor)

Once you relax, give yourself at least an equal amount of rest break time to make sure you feel your pelvic floor completely relaxing prior to doing your next Kegel. If you squeeze for four seconds, then rest for at least four seconds. Going back to our analogy, consciously bring the elevator down to the ground floor.

If initially you can only hold your Kegel for the sprint-time duration of two to four seconds, keep practicing until you build your endurance to hold for a longer duration. Five seconds is the minimum marathon-fiber duration, and you will want to keep practicing until you can reach a goal of ten seconds. Once you have mastered each type, alternate your practice so you are doing both sprints and marathons.

How Often to Kegel

How many Kegels should you do during the day? There is a huge variance in the suggested amount of Kegels to do for strengthening your pelvic floor, ranging from twenty-four to two hundred. I know if someone told me to do something two hundred times during the day, I wouldn't do any, because two hundred sounds way too overwhelming. I ask patients to do twenty-four Kegels a day because that seems like a feasible goal. Anything more than twenty-four Kegels is a bonus!

The *quality* of your Kegels should be your main guide as you determine how many repetitions to do. If your Kegels lack good quality, then your body is cheating and developing bad habits. Remember, you should be squeezing to engage your core and pelvic floor only. To help my patients avoid this cheating, I first see how many seconds they can hold a Kegel properly. Then I see how many repetitions they can do in a row, at that specific duration, with good technique before getting tired.

If you will put on your math cap for a minute, I will help you figure out how many you should do. Let's say you can properly hold the Kegel for four seconds and you can do five Kegels in a row (at four seconds) before getting tired. That means you need to do five rounds of five repetitions of Kegels throughout the day (twenty-five) to hit at least twenty-four, which is the daily goal. If instead you can do three Kegels in a row, then you need to do eight rounds of three repetitions throughout the day to hit twenty-four. Breaking it up into sets like this will ensure that you're isolating the correct muscle groups and not getting tired. As I mentioned, it's best to combine sprints and marathons. Your ultimate goal is to hold a ten-second Kegel for ten repetitions once a day and a two-second Kegel for ten repetitions once a day with an additional four more Kegels of your choice. This will give you a grand total of at least— you guessed it (or did the math)—twenty-four Kegels a day.

The Knack

We discussed the knack previously in chapter 4, "Bladder Health." Essentially, the knack is a Kegel that has impeccable timing. As you may recall, normally the pelvic floor muscles and core muscles will automatically squeeze just *prior* to coughing, sneezing, laughing, lifting, or any task that results in increased abdominal pressure. This automatic squeeze provides support to your internal organs so that the force produced by your pelvic floor muscles and core muscles is greater than the force produced in abdominal pressure from the task (sneezing or lifting). This results in a counterbrace that not only prevents bladder leakage, but also provides stabilization to your pelvic girdle, spine, and hips. To help refresh your memory, figure 42 shows the same illustration as figure 20.

Figure 42: Increased Abdominal Pressure on the Bladder Without and With the Knack

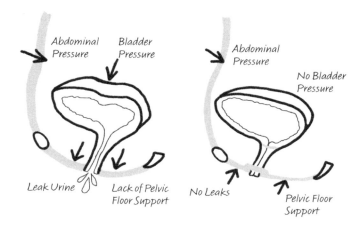

Try to remember: That split second you have when you're about to sneeze, squeeze! Prior to standing up, squeeze! The biggest challenge is remembering to do it. The good news? This can count as a Kegel repetition to help you reach your goal of twenty-four a day. As with Kegels, when you are done knacking, it is important to relax your pelvic floor muscles so they do not stay tense and tight. Your pelvic floor muscles should naturally do this, but it doesn't hurt to take a deep belly breath after doing the knack just to make sure!

Let Your Hips Help You Kegel

At the third layer of the pelvic floor, the obturator internus muscle has a special role. This muscle not only acts to support the pelvic girdle but also helps to stabilize the hip. Because of this, strengthening your hip muscles will help to strengthen your pelvic floor through what we call "overflow." Think of the muscle engagement of your hips overflowing to the neighboring muscle group: your pelvic floor. This is especially true if you do a Kegel during the hip-strengthening exercise.

For example, let's say you're doing squats, lunges, or a leg machine at the gym—any lower-extremity exercise. As you're working out, be sure to squeeze to engage your core and pelvic floor too! With that in mind, if your plan is to do twelve lunges, then you may need to take a standing rest break for a few seconds halfway through to give your pelvic floor a rest. It's a two-for-one here, ladies! And, if you do twelve squats and squeeze to engage your pelvic floor and core each time, then guess what? You just did twelve Kegels out of your goal for twenty-four a day.

Breathing is especially important to pay attention to when you're exercising. As we've discussed, using the Valsalva technique (holding your breath when lifting, straining, or exercising) is common but not recommended, because when you hold your breath, it places increased pressure through your abdominal and pelvic area. Instead, when you are exercising or lifting, think about exhaling during the squeezing part of the motion, which will always be the part that requires more exertion. For example, if you're doing a squat or a lunge, inhale when you're lowering toward the ground. When you're exerting yourself and squeezing up to stand, exhale. Remember too that when doing a Kegel, it is easiest to initiate while exhaling, so using the correct breathing pattern will also help remind you when to squeeze to engage your core and pelvic floor. Finally, I just have to add that if you're grunting or holding your breath with your eyeballs about to pop out of your head, then you should decrease the amount of weight you're lifting. Don't aim to impress others; gym and exercise time—like bathroom time!—is for YOU.

Core Isolation Exercises

As you will see, all of the core isolation exercises are performed lying down. Although you are ultimately improving your core, these "isolation" exercises actually begin by squeezing to engage both your core and your pelvic floor (which I describe in the instructions as *perform the knack*), because these muscles are best friends and work together. You will then hold the squeeze throughout each exercise.

Here are some more key points to keep in mind as you do these exercises:

- Breathe throughout the movement; do not hold your breath.
- Ensure your pelvis is in a neutral position where your low back is not excessively arched or pressed flat against the floor. There should be a small, natural curve of your low back against the floor.
- When moving your legs, keep your spine and pelvis neutral and still; do not let it arch upward or press into the ground. If you're not squeezing your core and pelvic floor well enough, your spine will want to move out of its neutral position.
- When moving your legs, keep your pelvis neutral and still; do not let it teeter-totter. If you're not squeezing your core and pelvic floor well enough, then when your leg moves, your pelvis will teeter to that side.
- You will want to perform these exercises to fatigue, which means that you should do as many repetitions as you can with good technique where your pelvis and spine stay still. Some women may be able to do four repetitions while others may be able to do fifteen repetitions. Each of the exercises is progressively more challenging. Progress to the next exercise only after you can do fifteen repetitions of one exercise with good technique. Aim to perform these exercises one to two times a day, progressing to up to fifteen repetitions.

Let's get moving!

Supine bent knee fall out (figure 43): Lie on your back with your knees bent and feet flat on the floor. Perform the knack and hold it while you let your right knee fall out to about a forty-five degree angle. Moving slowly and with control, return your right knee to the starting position. Release the knack so you can rest (if needed), then perform it again and repeat the exercise with your left leg.

Figure 43: Supine Bent Knee Fall Out

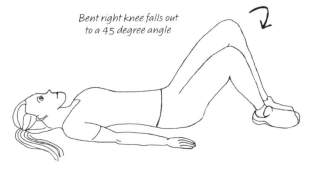

Bent right knee falls out to a 45 degree angle

Supine heel slide (figure 44): Lie on your back with your knees bent and feet flat on the floor. Perform the knack and slide your right heel so your right knee straightens. Return to the starting position by sliding your heel back up toward your butt. Release the knack so you can rest (if needed), then perform it again and repeat the exercise with your left leg.

Figure 44: Supine Heel Slide

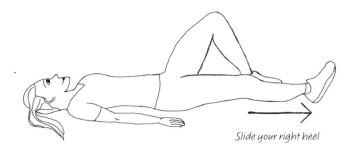

Slide your right heel

Supine march (figure 45)*:* Lie on your back with your knees bent and feet flat on the floor. Perform the knack and lift your right leg up as if you were marching. Your upper thigh will move to form a ninety-degree angle with your hip. Return your right marching leg down to the starting position, so your knee is bent and foot flat on the floor. Release the knack so you can rest (if needed), then perform it again and repeat the exercise with your left leg.

Figure 45: Supine March

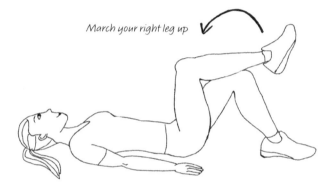

March your right leg up

Supine double march (figure 46): Lie on your back with your knees bent and feet flat on the floor. Perform the knack and lift one leg up as if you were marching. Your upper thigh will move to form a ninety-degree angle with your hip. March the other leg up to match. At this point, both legs will be lifted in a double march position. Return one leg down to the starting position, so your knee is bent and foot flat on the floor, followed by the other leg. Release the knack so you can rest (if needed), then perform it again and repeat the exercise.

Figure 46: Supine Double March

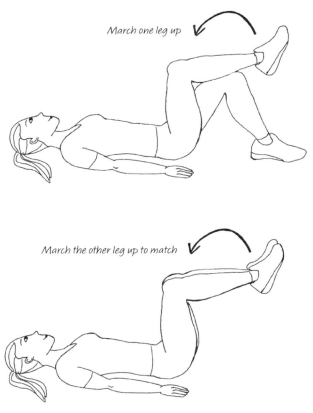

March one leg up

March the other leg up to match

Supine double up and double down (figure 47): Lie on your back with your knees bent and feet flat on the floor. Perform the knack and march both legs up at the same time. Your upper thighs will move to form a ninety-degree angle with your hips. Lower both legs down at the same time. Release the knack so you can rest (if needed), then perform it again and repeat the exercise.

Figure 47: Supine Double Up and Double Down

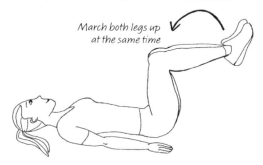

March both legs up
at the same time

Vaginal Weights

Vaginal weights are small circular or oval-shaped weights that are inserted vaginally to strengthen the pelvic floor muscles. They come in a set that progressively increases in weight, which is measured in grams, not pounds! For example, the smallest weight might be as light as a AA battery and the heaviest weight might be as heavy as an avocado. Vaginal weights, like pelvic floor muscle wands and dilators, can be ordered online. I personally recommend the Intimate Rose brand.

To use vaginal weights, start with the lightest one, insert it vaginally, and hold it in place by performing the knack. A warning: more often than not, your body will want to cheat when you are using these weights. You're supposed to use only your pelvic floor and core muscles, but it's easy to tilt your pelvis, squeeze your butt cheeks, and press your thighs together to help hold the weight in. To avoid this, you may want to try using the weights in the shower. If you are moving to wash your body or shave your legs, the movement may eliminate or reduce the cheating.

The research regarding vaginal weights is inconclusive when compared to doing pelvic floor muscle training, such as Kegels, alone,[20] so I'll let you be the judge! If you need to strengthen your pelvic floor, you can certainly give vaginal weights a try—just be sure to focus only on squeezing to engage only your core and pelvic floor!

Note to readers: The next two chapters discuss pregnancy and postpartum conditions and treatments. Although the narration is primarily focused on full-term pregnancies with healthy outcomes, I would like to take a moment to acknowledge that this may not be the case for all women. Pregnancy and postpartum issues may also affect women who experience miscarriages, terminations, surrogacy, premature births, stillbirths, infertility, and many other situations that can pose serious challenges to your mental, physical, and emotional health. If you are facing any of these situations, please know that I am truly sorry—having experienced a miscarriage myself, I understand how devastating these situations can be. It is very important for all women to make sure they get the services, treatment, and support they need. As a starting point, the resources in Appendix B may help.

CHAPTER EIGHT

Pregnancy

"A woman is the full circle.
Within her is the power to create,
nurture, and transform."

—Diane Mariechild

PREGNANCY CAUSES GREAT CHANGE for a woman's body. It is beautiful, challenging, emotional, and miraculous. For nine months, your body is on loan, nurturing your growing child. After delivery, your body is going through changes caring for your newborn, especially if you are breastfeeding.

Postpartum depression is three times higher in those with back or pelvic pain than those without pain.[21] In Europe, it is standard practice that women receive a referral to physical therapy during this timeframe. Unfortunately, that doesn't usually happen in the United States, where there is more of a misconception that any pain you are experiencing is normal or will go away with time, suggesting you have to "deal with it." However, it doesn't have to be this way! I want to emphasize that pain is NOT normal during pregnancy, and a woman should not be expected to carry out her pregnancy in pain. If a woman can have a relatively pain-free pregnancy *and* decrease her risk of postpartum depression, then it is a win-win situation and a no-brainer! Ask your doctor for a referral to physical therapy if you're having pregnancy-related pain (or any pain for that matter).

This chapter is designed to give you a brief overview of what happens not only between your hips but also throughout your whole body during pregnancy and how physical therapy can be critical during this time period. In the next sections, we'll review body changes, exercise, preparations for birth (learning how to push effectively), high-risk conditions, and labor and delivery (learning why delivering on your back is not ideal). As you will discover, a woman's body is just incredibly amazing. There is a lot going on during the labor and delivery process, and with your first baby, it can feel especially scary and intimidating. Working with a pelvic floor physical therapist can help you feel and be most prepared for this special time in your life. Let's get started!

BODY CHANGES

A woman's body goes through many changes during pregnancy to adapt and support the growing baby. Let's take a closer look at these changes.

Hormones

The following hormones all play an active role in pregnancy:

Estrogen increases the size of the breasts and uterus, and it relaxes ligaments and joints; estrogen levels increase up to thirty times during pregnancy.

Progesterone assists to relax the uterus and gastrointestinal system, contributing to pregnancy-related acid reflux and constipation. (See chapter 5, "Bowel Health," for ways to manage constipation.)

Prolactin promotes lactation and aids in milk production at the end of pregnancy.

Relaxin relaxes soft tissues and joints, prevents the expanding uterus from contracting during pregnancy, and softens the cervix.

Body Systems

The following body systems also play an active role during pregnancy.

Balance System

During pregnancy, the balance point, also known as center of gravity, of the body moves forward and up, accommodating your growing abdomen. Due to this change, 25 percent of pregnant women fall, and as a women progresses in her pregnancy, it gets harder to balance. Once postpartum, her balance will stay declined for another six to eight weeks.[22] The good news is that physical therapy can help new mothers retrain the core muscles and pelvic floor muscles to stabilize the spine, pelvis, and hips.

Cardiovascular System

Heart rate increases, as does the amount of blood the heart pumps. Blood pressure decreases because the blood vessels dilate and expand.[23]

Gastrointestinal System

Acid reflux and constipation may occur from hormonal changes that are causing relaxation of the gastrointestinal system.[24] Need I say it? Pelvic floor physical therapy for the win again!

Integumentary System

Stretch marks—own them! Stretch marks are most common over the lower abdomen but can also occur on your hips, thighs, breasts, and arms during pregnancy. Increased estrogen levels can contribute to blue star-shaped spider veins over your chest, arms, and legs. As far as hair and fingernails, every woman is different. Some will experience increased growth and stronger hair and fingernails, while others will experience hair loss and thinning fingernails.

Muscular System

The abdominal wall (which is where your core muscles sit), pelvic floor, and pelvic girdle are most affected. Here's how:

- Diastasis rectus abdominis (DRA) occurs when the rectus abdominis (the "six-pack" muscle) separates down the center as your baby grows, as shown in figure 48.
- There are increased demands placed on the pelvic floor to support the weight of the growing baby. During active labor, the pelvic floor muscles can stretch to three times their original resting length.[25]
- The pelvic girdle can be rotated or misaligned, contributing to pubic pain, low back pain, hip pain, coccyx pain, and/or sacroiliac joint pain. (See page 92 to learn how to address pelvic girdle alignment.) With hormone changes during pregnancy, there is increased joint and tissue laxity, which can contribute to pain and discomfort. In addition to ensuring that your pelvis is level, it is important to learn how to move and control your mobility within this extra range of motion and laxity. A physical therapist can assist with stabilization training to help your body better adjust to this.

Figure 48: Diastasis Rectus Abdominis

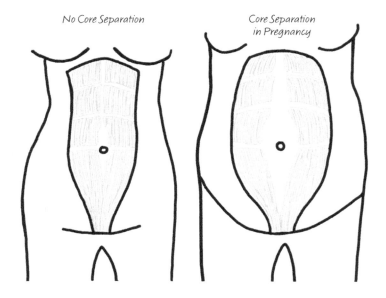

No Core Separation

Core Separation
in Pregnancy

Neurovascular System

Nerves are more likely to be compressed due to swelling from fluid retention. This commonly happens at the wrist, leading to carpal tunnel syndrome, and along the groin, leading to meralgia paresthetica, which is burning and tingling in the outer groin and thigh area. Meralgia paresthetica is also provoked from the increase in abdominal weight.[26] In both cases, numbness and/or tingling will occur in the palm of the hand and at the outer part of the upper thigh, respectively. I know you've guessed it—physical therapy, of course, can help with this!

Respiratory System

During pregnancy, the growing baby will restrict the diaphragm. This makes breathing more challenging, regardless of how much your rib cage widens to accommodate during your pregnancy.[27]

Renal System

As we've discussed, the kidneys constantly filter blood to remove waste and extra water, creating urine. During pregnancy, the total body water increases by eight liters, so the kidneys must work harder. As well, the bladder moves forward and up, making it harder to fully empty.[28] It is true that due to anatomical and physiological changes, during pregnancy a woman may have a change in bladder habits, but it is still not normal to leak or to have to pee every thirty minutes when pregnant. If this is you, consult a pelvic floor physical therapist.

Skeletal System

Due to hormonal changes, joints may become more relaxed, contributing to low back pain and/or pelvic pain. During pregnancy, the low back has an increased lordotic curve, and the arch of the foot may fall, causing the foot to lengthen. It is especially important to have the muscular strength and coordination to control your movements through the increase in joint mobility to minimize pain and discomfort.[29] Addressing your pelvic girdle alignment can help. Refer to page 92 of chapter 6, "Pelvic Pain."

Weight Gain

This is normal to support your growing baby. Average weight gain is thought to be twenty to thirty pounds. Half of the weight gained is due to the fetus, placenta, and amniotic fluid; a quarter is due to the uterus and breasts; and another quarter is due to maternal body fluid.[30] Although weight gain is normal, a 20 percent weight gain is thought to increase joint force by 100 percent.[31] This can contribute to pain and discomfort—all the more reason to consult a physical therapist.

EXERCISE

As you already know, when you exercise positive endorphins are released that help improve your mental well-being. This is still true during pregnancy. In general, exercise during pregnancy has many cardiovascular benefits, it can help decrease your risk of needing a c-section, and it can increase the placenta capacity.[32] As well, exercising before and during pregnancy can decrease the risk of developing preeclampsia. Regular exercise during the first twenty weeks of pregnancy decreases risk by greater than 40 percent. It is even thought that moderate to high weight-bearing exercise during pregnancy can lead to advanced neurodevelopment for the baby.[33]

The American College of Obstetricians and Gynecologists (ACOG) has published guidelines for exercise during the pregnancy and postpartum time period, and in this section we will review these guidelines and general recommendations.[34] Always consult your healthcare provider prior to starting an exercise routine and any time that questions arise as you implement it.

Additionally, it's important to add that because high-risk pregnancy can lead to serious conditions with many variations and restrictions, readers with high-risk pregnancy should consult directly with their healthcare providers and avoid all exercise unless they have their physician's approval. The following exercise guidelines do *not* apply to readers with high-risk pregnancy, which is discussed later in this chapter.

General Exercise Guidelines

Here are some general guidelines for exercise during pregnancy:

- Aim for thirty minutes of moderate intensity daily. Use the "talk test" to determine moderate intensity: you should be able to talk but not sing while exercising at this intensity.
- Avoid high-fall-risk activities and scuba diving.
- Avoid lying on your back, when exercising and sleeping, after the first trimester.
- Take caution with altitudes over 6,000 feet.

Note that when you are postpartum, exercise helps decrease risk for postpartum depression, and moderate weight loss while nursing is okay.

When to Avoid Exercise

Exercise is typically contraindicated (not allowed) with the following conditions:

- Heart/lung disease
- Incompetent cervix
- Persistent second- or third-trimester bleeding
- Placenta previa after twenty-six weeks gestation
- Preeclampsia/hypertension
- Preterm labor with current pregnancy
- Risk of preterm labor
- Ruptured membranes
- Severe anemia

When to Stop Exercise

If you experience these signs and symptoms while exercising, stop immediately and seek medical attention.

- Amniotic fluid leak or vaginal bleeding
- Calf pain, which indicates a risk for blood clots (deep vein thrombosis)
- Chest pain

- Decreased fetal movements
- Dizziness
- Shortness of breath before exertion
- Headache
- Muscle weakness
- Preterm labor

Examples of Suitable Exercise

The mode of exercise can vary significantly as long as you are following the guidelines. Here are a few great suggestions:

- Dancing
- Modified yoga
- Resistance training
- Rowing
- Stationary cycling
- Swimming
- Walking and jogging
- Hiking

Body Mechanics and Movement

As your unborn baby grows, it is important to be mindful of how you're moving your body. With a diastasis rectus abdominis (DRA) and lengthening of your pelvic floor, you may find that your abdomen, spine, and hips become weak and painful. When doing any movement, you can help yourself by using the following tips to improve your body mechanics.

- Squeeze to engage your pelvic floor and core by doing the knack prior to any exertion like coughing, sneezing, laughing, lifting, or standing. This step helps to give you added support and stability to your spine, hips, and pelvic organs.
- Keep your pelvis neutral and spine long. When standing, lifting, or carrying, ensure your low back is in a neutral position where it is not excessively arched forward or flattened. There should be a small, natural curve in your low back. When your pelvis and spine

are in this position, you can better squeeze to engage your core and pelvic floor to improve your overall stability.

- Be aware of your knees. When standing, sitting, lifting, or climbing stairs, make sure your knees stay in line with your feet and hips. If your knees fall in toward each other, you are not adequately using your hips to stabilize, and this can lead to knee and hip discomfort.

Additionally, please refer to the "Core Isolation Exercises" on page 113. These exercises will show you how to strengthen your abdominal wall and help generate force to stabilize your spine and pelvis, especially if you have a DRA during pregnancy.

Again, it is imperative to discuss exercise programs with your healthcare provider to determine what is best for you. In the absence of a high-risk pregnancy, exercise is recommended and encouraged. Our bodies are designed to move and be active, even when pregnant.

PREPARING YOURSELF FOR BIRTH

In addition to all of the exciting and happy feelings pregnancy can bring, it also includes fear, anxiety, and uncertainty with what the future holds. Will you have a vaginal or c-section delivery? Will your pelvic floor tear during delivery if you deliver vaginally? How will your body handle the pain? Will you try a natural route or ask for an epidural? Every woman's pregnancy, labor, and delivery experience is different and unique, and we should not compare ourselves to others. With that in mind, there are a few things that you can do to be proactive to help set you up to be more comfortable during the labor and delivery period. It is again important to mention that because high-risk pregnancy is a serious condition with many variations and restrictions, readers with a high-risk pregnancy should consult directly with their healthcare providers to ensure that the following strategies are safe to begin.

Pelvic Girdle Alignment

It is important to address pelvic girdle alignment during pregnancy and prior to delivery. As you know, when the pelvis is properly aligned, your pelvic floor muscles can do their job better; they can better provide support during pregnancy and lengthen during delivery. If your pelvic girdle is rotated, then the pelvic floor muscles follow suit, which may contribute to increased risk of perineal tearing, discomfort, and prolonged recovery. See page 92 for instructions for the pelvic correction.

Perineal Massage

Perineal massage is a stretch done to the pelvic floor muscles and perineal tissue six weeks prior to your due date to decrease risk of perineal trauma—such as tearing or the need for an episiotomy—during vaginal delivery. Research suggests that this is most effective for those who have never given birth vaginally, but perineal massage can also help decrease postpartum perineal pain for those who have previously delivered vaginally.[35] A pelvic floor physical therapist can perform this for you and teach you and/or your partner how to perform it. You (or your partner) will want to perform the massage for up to ten minutes once a day. Those of you who are go-getters and want to do more than ten minutes, there is no need! The key is to try to stretch for a short period of time (ten minutes) every day versus a longer period of time (thirty minutes) only a few times a week. Be sure to wash your hands prior to starting the massage, and always use lubrication.

To stretch, lie on your back with your knees bent and supported with pillows so your legs can relax. Insert your thumb (or have your partner insert a finger) vaginally. If your tailbone position is at 6:00 and your pubic bone position is at 12:00, then stretch by pressing down from 3:00 to 6:00 and 6:00 to 9:00, as shown in figure 49. Stretch the tissue until it gets taut, at which point you will feel pressure or a stretching feeling. If it is painful, use less pressure.

If you do experience perineal tearing or an episiotomy during delivery, do not stress! We will cover this topic in chapter 9, "Postpartum: The Fourth Trimester."

Learning How to Push

How exactly should you push during labor and delivery? This is a great topic for discussion because many women have never been taught how to

Figure 49: Perineal Stretching

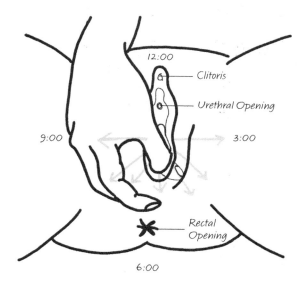

correctly push. Pushing via a Valsalva technique (basically, breath-holding-pushing-so-hard-your-eyeballs-might-pop-out) can causes the following:

- An increase in pelvic floor pressure, increasing the risk of pelvic organ prolapse
- An increase in abdominal pressure, increasing the risk for further abdominal wall separation with a diastasis rectus abdominis (DRA)
- Hemorrhoids
- Added exhaustion during labor and delivery
- Reflexive tightening of your pelvic floor muscles versus lengthening to stretch

Other delivery-related risk factors for pelvic organ prolapse include vacuum-assisted or forceps-assisted delivery and sustaining a perineal tear. See chapter 2, "When Your Pelvic Support System Fails," for further information on POP.

When pushing during delivery, try to use an open-glottis technique where you exhale forcefully during the pushing phase versus holding your breath. (A great time to practice this in advance is during a bowel movement.) When delivering a baby vaginally, your muscles need to lengthen to allow your baby to pass through the vaginal canal. This process obviously is painful, and your body's natural response may be to reflexively tighten your pelvic floor to guard and protect you from the pain. However, if your body is reflexively tightening your pelvic floor when you are trying to push, there can be an increased risk of perineal tearing. Even though this open-glottis pushing technique is what's recommended, everyone has a unique experience and you may need to hold your breath and grunt out those last few pushes. A pelvic floor physical therapist can work with you on coordinating your breathing and teach you pushing strategies that allow you to remain aware of relaxing through your pelvic floor.

HIGH-RISK PREGNANCY CONDITIONS[36]

As noted, high-risk pregnancy can lead to serious conditions with many variations and restrictions. Consequently, readers with high-risk pregnancy should consult directly with their healthcare providers and avoid all exercise unless they have their physician's approval. This section is intended to serve as an overview only.

High-risk pregnancy occurs with conditions such as the following:

- Hypertension (HTN), which is another term for high blood pressure
- Incompetent cervix
- Intrauterine growth restriction (IUGR)
- Placenta previa
- Preterm labor
- Gestational diabetes mellitus (GDM)
- Transient osteoporosis

This section explores each of these issues in more detail and then describes ways you may find yourself working with a physical therapist while you are being monitored.

Hypertension (HTN)

There are four ways to categorize HTN in pregnancy:

1. *Chronic:* high blood pressure prior to pregnancy.
2. *Gestational:* blood pressure increases during pregnancy but resolves twelve weeks postpartum.
3. *Preeclampsia:* blood pressure increases after twenty weeks gestation, prior to which it was normal; protein is found in the urine; and blood pressure is >140/>90. With severe preeclampsia, blood pressure is >160/>110.
4. *Eclampsia:* central nervous system failure; it presents the same as preeclampsia, with the addition of seizures.

Preeclampsia is associated with an inflammatory immune system response and affects many body systems, including the blood and blood vessels, liver, kidney, and nervous system. With preeclampsia, the placenta can develop lesions much like that of atherosclerosis. Symptoms of preeclampsia include the following:

- Swelling of the arms and legs
- Headache
- Heartburn
- Right-sided rib cage pain
- Visual field flashing lights

Incompetent Cervix

The cervix is the lower part of the uterus that meets the top part of the vaginal canal. Normally, the cervix is closed firmly, but as pregnancy progresses, it softens and dilates (opens). Incompetent cervix is when the cervix softens and dilates early, during the second or third trimester, leading to risk of preterm birth.

Intrauterine Growth Restriction (IUGR)

Intrauterine growth restriction occurs when the overall growth of the baby and the baby's organs are restricted. IUGR can be a result of several factors, including the following:

- Fetal factors: birth defects, chromosomal abnormalities, infection, multiple babies (twins or triplets)
- Maternal factors: alcohol or drug abuse, high blood pressure, infection, kidney disease, malnutrition
- Uterus/placenta factors: decreased blood flow, infection, placenta detachment from the uterus, placenta previa (see next section)

Placenta Previa

The placenta normally attaches to the top or side wall of the uterus, connecting to your baby via the umbilical cord. The placenta and umbilical cord supply oxygen and nutrients to your baby. Placenta previa occurs when the placenta attaches over or near the cervix. There are four stages outlined below and shown in figure 50:

Stage I: Low lying indicates the placenta is at the lower uterine segments.

Stage II: Marginal indicates the edge of the placenta is at the margin of internal cervix.

Stage III: Partial indicates the internal cervix is partially covered.

Stave IV: Total indicates the internal cervix is totally covered.

With Stage III and Stage IV, the placenta can separate from the uterine wall, leading to hemorrhaging and risk for preterm birth. If placenta previa does not resolve, it will usually result in a c-section delivery.

Preterm Labor

Preterm labor results with the onset of labor prior to thirty-seven weeks gestation. It can result from many of the previously mentioned factors. Symptoms of preterm labor include the following:

- Backaches
- Cramping or contractions

Figure 50: Stages of Placenta Previa

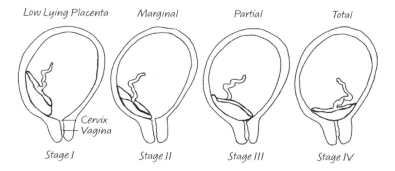

Low Lying Placenta   Marginal   Partial   Total

Cervix
Vagina

Stage I   Stage II   Stage III   Stage IV

- Vaginal discharge, bleeding, or having your water break
- Vaginal or pelvic pressure

Gestational Diabetes Mellitus (GDM)

Testing for GDM occurs at twenty-four to twenty-eight weeks gestation. Risk factors for developing GDM include a sedentary lifestyle, obesity, and increased maternal age. Signs of GDM include the following:

- Abnormal urine tests
- Excessive thirst
- Fatigue
- Frequent urination
- Infections
- Nausea
- Changes in vision, such as blurred vision

GDM can result in larger-birthweight babies, preterm labor and delivery, increased chance of c-section delivery, and adverse health for your baby. Management includes dietary modifications, regular exercise, and insulin if needed.

Transient Osteoporosis

Transient osteoporosis occurs from an increase in calcium demand resulting in bone loss from the mother's skeleton during the pregnancy or early postpartum period, especially if breastfeeding. It is reversible, lasting two to twelve months postpartum, and the spine and hips are most commonly affected. Symptoms include a sudden onset of pain and loss of mobility within the affected area.[37]

Physical Therapy Support During Monitoring of High-Risk Pregnancy

With a high-risk pregnancy, the goal is to decrease abdominal pressure and uterine contractions. A specific exercise program is contraindicated (not allowed) during this time. If you are admitted to the hospital for monitoring, then physical therapy, which should be provided during your stay, will offer specific steps to support you with the following:

- Bed mobility and transfer training
- Breathing strategies and avoiding the Valsalva maneuver (breath holding and straining with exertion)
- Coordination of pelvic floor muscles and core muscles for ease of delivery
- Decreasing emotional stress
- Decreasing risk for pressure sores, skin break down, and deconditioning side effects of bed rest
- Maintaining the strength and function of your musculoskeletal system
- Facilitating uterine blood flow via a left-side lying position
- Relaxation strategies

LABOR AND DELIVERY

Labor consists of three different stages—pre-labor, active labor, and transition—followed by delivery. Understanding what happens during each stage, along with identifying the best position to deliver in, will help you through this process. Let's take a look at the details surrounding labor and delivery.

Stages of Labor

The experiences in each stage of labor are different for everyone. However, the following descriptions will give you a general idea of what to expect:[38]

- *Pre-labor:* Fifteen-second contractions that are ten to thirty minutes apart. During this stage, membranes rupture and the cervix thins, which can lead to bloody discharge. Cervical dilation is around three centimeters.
- *Active labor:* Forty-five-second contractions that are two to five minutes apart. Cervical dilation is around six centimeters. This stage can last up to five hours with your first baby.
- *Transition:* Ninety-second contractions that are one to two minutes apart. Cervical dilation is around eight to ten centimeters. The stretch receptors of the levator ani muscle group (the third layer of the pelvic floor muscles) activate, resulting in an urge to push.

Birthing Positions

Did you know that the traditional delivery position of lying on your back, legs spread wide with your feet in stirrups, is usually not the best position for you? This traditional approach is now thought to increase the stress and tension placed on your pelvic floor.[39] As we've discussed in other chapters, your pelvic floor muscles attach to your tailbone, which naturally moves a little bit (five to twenty-five degrees to be exact). If you are lying on your back, then your tailbone and pelvic floor muscles may be restricted against the bed. You can certainly labor when lying on your back if you wish to do so, but ideally you should move to a different position when it comes time to push. If possible, perform your pushing—and thus delivery—in one of the following positions.

Side-lying delivery position (figure 51): Lie on either side so your top leg is pulled up toward you where your hip and knee are bent. Your bent knee will be pointing toward the ceiling to further open up your pelvic floor. You can hold your leg up with your top arm, but likely your partner, nurse, or labor support person will need to help you—especially if you have an epidural.

Figure 51: Side-Lying Delivery Position

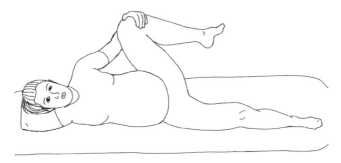

Tabletop delivery position (figure 52): In this modified yoga-style position, you are on your hands and knees. You will want to ensure that your knees and thighs are spread a little bit wider than the standard tabletop position, to further open up your pelvic floor. If you need more support, you can use a stack of pillows or an exercise ball under your chest and arms.

Figure 52: Tabletop Delivery Position

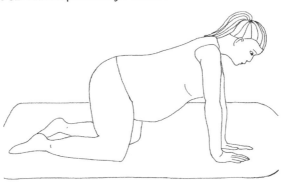

Supported squat delivery position (figure 53): For this position you will need a squat bar (no—not like what is in a gym). In this case, a squat bar is an arching handrail attached to the bed. You are in a deep squat position with your knees and feet wide. Your upper body is resting on the squat bar for added support.

Figure 53: Supported Squat Delivery Position

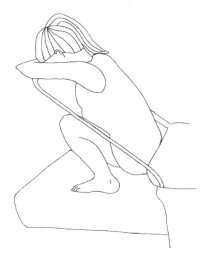

Upright and lateral positions, such as the ones illustrated, can decrease perineal trauma.[40] Specifically, upright positions allow the pelvis to better expand during delivery and utilize the effects of gravity to assist with delivery.[41] At this point you might be wondering, "Why, then, have so many women been lying on their back for delivery for all these years?" The answer: it is easiest for the doctor to deliver the baby when you are in this position. However, your doctor is capable of helping deliver your baby in any position!

There are certain situations when you may not be able to—or when you may not choose to—use an alternate position. The first is with a vacuum-assisted or forceps-assisted delivery, in which case the goal is to deliver the baby quickly and you need to be positioned where your doctor can best use these delivery assistive devices (usually this will be on your back). The second is when lying on your back is in fact the most comfortable position for you and is where you can generate your best push. Because everyone is unique, maybe you prefer your back—and that is okay! The bottom line is to understand that you have options for the position you deliver in.

Determining your optimal delivery positioning is especially helpful if you are experiencing any back, hip, tailbone, or pelvic pain. As noted, a physical therapist can meet with you in advance to help determine which birthing position might be best for you and to practice coordinating your breathing to help you generate your best, most effective push.

Delivery

There are two methods of delivery: vaginal or c-section. This section briefly explores the unique benefits and challenges of each method.

Vaginal Delivery

With a vaginal delivery, the delivery process begins once you are ten centimeters dilated. Remember, during labor and delivery the pelvic floor muscles stretch up to three times their normal resting length! This takes time because the muscles must gradually stretch to this length to decrease risk of tearing.

During the transition stage of labor, as mentioned earlier, the receptors of the levator ani muscles activate, creating an urge to push. Without an epidural, you will feel an urge to push. With an epidural, the urge to push may or may not be present. If there is no urge to push, then pushing should be delayed until the baby's head is visible, indicating that the levator ani's stretch receptors are activated for pushing. Remember that when you are pushing, you have positional options (side lying, tabletop, or a supported squat), and you can lie on your back between contractions to rest.

As babies move through the vaginal canal, they come in contact with extra-protective vaginal fluid and bacteria, which is generally thought to help establish healthy gut bacteria to decrease risk of asthma, allergies, and immune disorders.

C-Section Delivery

With a c-section, the surgeon will need to cut several layers of tissue to deliver the baby from the uterus. Since the baby does not pass through the vaginal canal, there is no risk of vaginal tearing or the need for an episiotomy: a big pro. However, your baby does not come in contact with the extra-protective vaginal fluid and bacteria mentioned above. To address this potential concern, some doctors use a technique called vaginal seeding, which involves using gauze to swab the vaginal canal and then transfer the fluid onto the newborn baby's skin, mouth, and nose. At this time, however, the long-term benefits of vaginal seeding is unclear. Also, due to the risk of transferring vaginal infections such as herpes, chlamydia, and gonorrhea from mom to baby, the American College of Obstetricians and Gynecologists recommend that vaginal seeding should only be done in a research setting.[42] If you do expect to have a c-section delivery, then this topic may be worth a discussion with your doctor; you never know if the doctor is participating in a research study or if this would be a safe option for you!

Cord Clamping

Once your baby is delivered vaginally or via c-section, the umbilical cord must be clamped and cut. The umbilical cord connects the baby to the placenta and is responsible for transferring oxygen-rich blood and nutrients from mom to baby. The American College of Obstetricians and Gynecologists recommend delayed cord clamping for at least thirty to sixty seconds after birth for both term and preterm infants.[43] Delayed cord clamping can provide your baby with added oxygen-rich blood flow to improve iron stores and developmental outcomes. It is important to discuss delayed cord clamping with your healthcare providers in advance and understand that even though this approach is recommended, it may not always be utilized. For example, if your baby is born emergently and needs immediate medical attention, the cord will likely be cut right away in order to provide other medical services to your baby.

Afterbirth

Once your baby is delivered and the umbilical cord is clamped and cut, the remainder of the umbilical cord and placenta, along with any other afterbirth, must be delivered. With a c-section, the doctor will manually remove this from your uterus. With a vaginal delivery, afterbirth delivery can happen spontaneously, or it can be manually removed.

Fundal Massage

This is an imperative uterine massage done after delivery to help the uterus contract to decrease bleeding, to remove excess blood, and to help pass any clots. Don't be fooled; this "massage" can be quite painful. If bleeding does not resolve with the fundal massage, additional measures will be taken as recommended by your doctor.

CHAPTER NINE

Postpartum: The Fourth Trimester

"Postpartum is a quest back to yourself.
Alone in your body again.
You will never be the same,
you are stronger than you were."

—Amethyst Joy

YOU JUST GAVE BIRTH to a beautiful baby, or babies! This new, precious human is depending on you and your partner for feeding, changing, protecting, and loving. But what about you? What about the fact that you hurt, your body just gave birth, and it needs to recover? You're tired because you labored for a day—or days—and haven't slept a wink, and now you are up during the night taking care of your baby. What about the emotional adjustment of having someone so dependent on you, Mom? It is scary! You cannot give from an empty cup, so it is essential that you take care of yourself and your needs during this time and in the years to come!

Just as physical therapy can help during pregnancy, it can also assist with healing during the postpartum time frame. It's important to touch on a few specific points regarding postpartum expectations.

Even with a c-section delivery, women can experience urinary incontinence because these women still experienced the hormonal changes and the downward pressure of carrying their baby during pregnancy. As I've mentioned before, I cannot tell you how many times I've heard women say, "Well, my doctor told me it was normal to leak because I've had children." Remember: this is NOT normal, and you do not need to live with this. Right after giving birth you *may* leak, since your body is still going through an incredible change. However, once you've reached six weeks postpartum and your body has had time to heal, it's time to get down to business and get the leaking taken care of.

Contrary to what most people think, leaking after childbirth is not always due to weak pelvic floor muscles. I find that this is just as commonly due to tight, painful muscles, especially with any perineal tearing. It is important to address the coordination and sequencing of pelvic floor muscle and core muscle contractions to lift and support the bladder. See page 50 for review on urinary incontinence and page 111 for review on the knack.

Sometimes, perineal tearing will extend into the external anal sphincter muscle, and fecal incontinence can become a concern. Vacuum-assisted and forceps-assisted deliveries also contribute to fecal incontinence if there is damage to the anal sphincter muscles. Like urinary incontinence, this can be due to weak or tight pelvic floor muscles; in any case, it is not normal. Refer back to page 81 for more information on fecal incontinence.

Pelvic pain can be present postpartum regardless of the type of birth you had. Like urinary incontinence, it is not EVER normal to have pelvic pain—babies or not and perineal tearing or not! See chapter 6, "Pelvic Pain," for further discussion.

A pelvic floor physical therapist can work with you to identify your specific needs regarding postpartum care for bladder health, bowel health, and pelvic pain. You can begin pelvic floor physical therapy immediately postpartum, but an internal pelvic floor muscle assessment (discussed in chapter 6, on page 91) cannot be performed until you are six weeks postpartum to allow your body time to heal. Once the assessment can take place, the therapist can determine if your pelvic floor muscles need to be lengthened or strengthened first.

Do not accept childbirth as a cause for a new "normal" that is incredibly *abnormal* when there are treatment options! Let's delve into more topics about postpartum care.

C-SECTION DELIVERY RECOVERY

If you deliver via c-section, the scar tissue on your lower abdomen will need to be massaged. Just like scar tissue anywhere in the body, if it does not get massaged, it can develop into restricting, painful, adhesions. Once the incision is healed and your doctor clears you, usually around the six-week mark, you can begin scar tissue massage. There is no wrong way to massage a scar: just rub it, move it, and stretch it! The fascia system, which is comprised of all layers of connective tissue, need to be able to glide and slide over each other and in all directions. Therefore, when you rub over your scar, you can glide the tissue right, left, in circles, in diagonal patterns, and so forth; any way works (see figure 54).

If you find that rubbing over the scar without any lotion is too uncomfortable, use a dab of scent-free lotion or Vitamin E oil to decrease the friction. If massaging is still too uncomfortable, simply stroke the scar with light pressure only (no massaging) to begin desensitizing it. You can use your fingertips, a tissue, a clean makeup brush, or anything else that will provide a light-textured touch to stroke the scar to decrease sensitivity. Practice these desensitization strategies (if needed) prior to progressing to scar massage. The massage itself should be done for five to ten minutes once a day until you feel the scar moves without restriction and is no longer sensitive or painful.

You will also want to practice diaphragmatic breathing (belly breathing) to treat your scar. When you inhale your breath deep into your belly, it assists to stretch and lengthen through the scar tissue. For review on this technique, refer to page 98.

Figure 54: C-Section Scar Massage Instructions

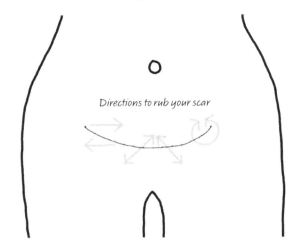

Directions to rub your scar

VAGINAL DELIVERY RECOVERY

If you deliver vaginally and have a perineal tear from tearing spontaneously or from an episiotomy, the scar tissue at the perineum will need to be massaged. Perineal tearing is graded as follows:

- *First degree:* tearing of the skin superficially
- *Second degree:* tearing of the skin superficially, plus tearing of the first layer of pelvic floor muscles
- *Third degree:* tearing of the skin superficially, tearing of the first layer of pelvic floor muscles, plus tearing of the perineal body and external anal sphincter muscle around the rectum
- *Fourth degree:* tearing of the skin superficially, tearing of the first layer of pelvic floor muscles, tearing of the perineal body and external anal sphincter muscle around the rectum, plus tearing into the pelvic diaphragm (third layer of pelvic floor muscles) and rectal mucosa

With tearing, your body creates scar tissue, which will require massaging. If you don't massage the perineal scar, you can experience pain with intercourse as well as bowel and bladder issues such as incontinence, because the pelvic floor muscles cannot optimally function with taut, tight scar tissue. Scar massage can be done once your incision is fully healed and your doctor clears you to do so, which is usually around the six-week mark.

This scar massage is similar to the perineal massage on page 130 and is done by inserting a lubricated thumb vaginally (after washing your hands, of course). You will be able to feel the scar tissue because it will feel more tight, taut, and even uncomfortable. When massaging the scar, you can move your thumb in any direction (e.g., in/out, right/left, in small circles, or pressing straight down)—anything to help stretch over and around the scar. Try to massage the scar for up to ten minutes a day. Inserting a vaginal dilator or using a pelvic floor muscle wand to further release the scar tissue can be of help too; refer to page 100 for review.

Once you no longer have pain with intercourse and daily tasks, you may stop performing the scar massage. You may find, however, that you need to perform this massage for a few minutes prior to intercourse to improve comfort. Physical therapy can provide specific guidance on this as well.

BREASTFEEDING AND YOUR PELVIC FLOOR

Believe it or not, breastfeeding affects your vaginal tissue. When breastfeeding, estrogen levels drop lower than they would drop if you didn't breastfeed.[44] Consequently, breastfeeding can further contribute to vaginal dryness and irritation. To address this, your gynecologist can prescribe topical creams during this time period.

When breastfeeding, your body needs an extra five hundred calories per day, and light to moderate exercise is encouraged.[45] In fact, light to moderate exercise for as long as ninety minutes typically will not affect your milk production as long as your caloric intake is adequate to meet the increase in energy demands. High-intensity exercise, on the other hand, may affect your milk supply,[46] so you may want to postpone that until your child is weaned.

Figure 55: Engaged Transverse Abdominis to Stabilize
Through a DRA

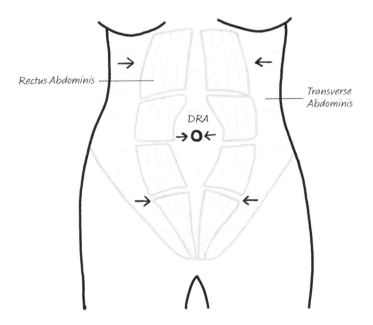

HEALING YOUR CORE

As mentioned earlier, the rectus abdominis muscle may separate during pregnancy, causing a diastasis rectus abdominis (DRA). A DRA occurs when the linea alba (the tissue connecting the right and left side of the "six-pack muscle") separates.

If you have a DRA, you may observe some doming (or bulging) down the middle of your belly. You can check the degree of the DRA by lying flat on your back with your knees bent so your feet are flat on the floor. Lift your head up off the floor while exhaling (breathing out) and use your fingertips to press over your belly button, moving your fingertips right and left until you can feel the more firm edges of the muscle. Normally, this distance will be less than or equal to two fingerbreadths. If it is greater than two finger breaths, it just means your core is separated a bit. This may or may not close, but that is okay! It is not the distance of separation that matters but rather your ability to stabilize and generate force through this separation to support your spine, hips, and pelvis. So just how do we do this? Well, do you remember what the most important core muscle is to help stabilize and ensure optimal pelvic health? Drum roll please . . . the transverse abdominis! This muscle wraps around the trunk like a corset would, so when you squeeze to engage your core, it draws the separated rectus abdominis muscle together and helps to generate tension through this point of weakness, as shown in figure 55.

Again, I would like to point out that it is OKAY if the separation does not close, but you will want to be able to stabilize through this area. To do this, please refer to the "Core Isolation Exercises" on page 113. You can begin core isolation exercises immediately postpartum; you do not need to postpone or delay them. These exercises will show you how to generate the force you need through the doming to try to assist with closing, which is just a bonus.

Once you have a foundation for working specifically on your core, let's take a look at how you can begin to use this strength functionally throughout your day. A convenient, functional exercise is a chair squat (figure 56). Here's how it works:

1. Start by sitting at the edge of a chair with your feet hip-width apart.
2. Squeeze to engage your core and your pelvic floor (just like you did in the core isolation exercises).
3. Continuing the squeeze, stand up. Keep your knees in line with your feet and hips; do not let them fall in toward your midline as you stand.
4. At the top of the stand, add in squeezing your butt cheek muscles and hold for two to three seconds.
5. Relax your core, pelvic floor, and butt cheek muscles and slowly return to the starting position sitting at the edge of the chair. As you return to sitting, keep your knees in line with your feet and hips; do not let them fall in toward your midline as you sit.
6. Repeat up to fifteen times. If you want more of a challenge, do this as you hold your baby!

Figure 56: Chair Squat

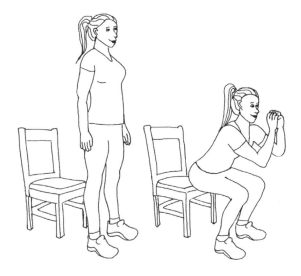

Additionally, you can (and should) squeeze to engage your core and pelvic floor while doing any daily task. Examples might include lifting your baby, carrying the car seat, lugging around diaper bags, or bringing in the groceries. Also squeeze to engage when getting in and out of the car and the bed, while doing dishes, folding laundry . . . any time of the day when you are exerting yourself!

Here are some key points to keep in mind as you use your core and pelvic floor functionally throughout the day:

- Remember to breathe while squeezing to engage your core and pelvic floor with chair squats and daily tasks, especially lifting tasks where breath holding may be more common.
- Utilize good body mechanics so that you stand close to the objects (and kiddos) you are lifting, lift from a squat position bending your legs, keep objects (and kiddos) close to you while carrying them, and of course, squeeze to engage your core and pelvic floor to give you extra strength and stability.

- Maintain neutral alignment (as we say in the PT world). This means being mindful of keeping your spine long and tall and keeping your knees in line with your hips and feet to create a strong, sturdy base to support you.

STRENGTHENING YOUR PELVIC FLOOR

You will also want to take steps to address your pelvic floor muscle strength as part of your postpartum recovery. As you perform the core exercises described in the previous section, your pelvic floor will also be squeezing to engage to assist. (Remember, the core and pelvic floor muscles are codependent.) However, prior to beginning more intense and specific pelvic floor muscle strengthening, such as Kegels, it is imperative to identify if your muscles need to be lengthened first. The gold standard would be to have a pelvic floor physical therapist assess your pelvic floor muscles once you are six weeks postpartum to guide you through this process. In the meantime, you can head on over to chapter 7, "To Lengthen or Strengthen" to read more about this matter. After reading this chapter, if you feel that your pelvic floor muscles are ready for strengthening, then you may begin Kegels. If you need more time to work on lengthening, that is completely okay. Take the time you need to lengthen your pelvic floor muscles and then begin strengthening at a later time; this approach will be more effective and productive in the long run.

RETURNING TO HIGH-LEVEL EXERCISE AND SPORTS

Now that we have covered some of the basics on immediate postpartum recovery, we should talk about the next step, which is returning to high-level exercise and sports. This looks different for everyone, depending on interest. Maybe you enjoy going for walks or playing golf or tennis. Maybe your goal is to compete in triathlons again, run races, or participate in exercise classes at your gym. Whatever your choice of exercise is, I highly recommend consulting a pelvic floor physical therapist to help guide you back into active participation. This professional guidance can decrease your risk of injury, help you understand appropriate exercise dosing, and teach you exercises to build appropriate strength and endurance so you can comfortably participate in the exercises of your choice. Best of all, it will help ensure that you have optimal pelvic function throughout it all.

POSTPARTUM DEPRESSION

Before we end the chapter, I want to add a few words about postpartum depression. It can be hard for people to truly understand the crippling effects of depression unless they have gone through it.

Risks of postpartum depression include having a prior history of depression, lack of social support, chronic health conditions, social isolation, and life stressors. A temporary, manageable case of "the baby blues"—mood swings, anxiety, irritability, and lack of sleep—is different than depression. With depression, the symptoms of the "baby blues" are scaled up and further include difficulty bonding with your baby, withdrawing from friends and family, feeling hopeless, and experiencing suicidal thoughts. *If you are experiencing suicidal thoughts, seek immediate medical attention.*

You do not need to be ashamed about any of these feelings, and you don't have to wear a "tough mama" badge. It is okay—and encouraged—to discuss these thoughts and feelings with your friends, family, and healthcare providers so you can get the help you need. This is a huge adjustment period, and you don't need to battle it alone. As hard as it may be, going for a walk or doing some form of gentle exercise can also help.

Talk about your feelings often. Postpartum depression affects one in nine mothers[47] and usually presents one to three weeks after delivery, although it can hit up to a year after.[48] I worked with a woman who developed her postpartum depression the day, *the day*, her baby was born. She recognized something was wrong because she didn't even want to hold her baby. However, instead of recognizing her depression, her providers made her feel ashamed and embarrassed of her behavior. Half the battle is recognizing the signs and understanding that you cannot take care of your baby if you are not healthy yourself.

CHAPTER TEN

Life Stages and Pelvic Health

"One day you will look back and see that all along, you were blooming."

—Morgan Harper Nichols

I N THIS CHAPTER, we will discuss the life stages of a woman— adolescence, reproductive years, menopause, and elderhood—in relationship to pelvic health. Much of this material also appeared in the previous chapters, so this will be a quick summary, with some additional woman-specific, life-stage changes to consider. I hope this chapter sheds even more light on how truly amazing a woman's body is and helps promote continued self-love at all ages.

Please note that females who are sexually active *at any age* may be at risk for sexually transmitted diseases. If you fall into that category, you will also want to read about testing in the bonus chapter, "Wellness Screening and Testing," and discuss your situation with your healthcare provider.

ADOLESCENCE

Even if you have put adolescence far behind you, please don't skip this section. This conversation will help you understand your own health as well as help you guide other females down this path—whether it be as a parent, family member, or mentor. If we can look out for each other and support each other in times of struggle, then maybe we can slowly pave a better way for women of all ages to learn to love themselves for who they are.

Despite the stereotypical image of "sweet sixteen," adolescence can pose a number of challenges. There is a lot of pressure placed on young girls, especially in regards to body image. Typically, the adolescent years are when females first become aware of societal pressure regarding body image. For some, this is an adolescent stage that can be overcome as they age and become more confident in their womanhood. However, some women can continue to carry unhealthy expectations into adulthood. I hope that women of all ages can confidently realize how silly and ridiculous these image expectations are. YOU are worth more. If you're worried about what other people think of you, learn to not care! Rachel Hollis wrote, "Someone else's opinion of you is none of your business."[49] If you feel you're losing control of some aspect of your life, don't try to regain it by making unhealthy diet and exercise choices. Reach out for support from a trusted friend, medical advisor such as a counselor, or family member.

In addition to facing emotional challenges, teen girls also face a variety of physical challenges. Did you know that adolescence is a vital time for bone formation and skeletal maturity for women? If a young woman has an eating disorder or is not getting a regular period during this time, then her skeletal system suffers, putting her at risk for osteopenia and osteoporosis. Additionally, 28 percent of collegiate female athletes experience stress urinary incontinence, with 40 percent of these women first noticing symptoms beginning in high school.[50] Don't be fooled; leaking doesn't just happen after a woman has had babies or as a woman gets older. What happens during these adolescent years can affect a girl for the rest of her life. In this section we will discuss the changes that occur with puberty and the importance of the menstrual cycle on bone formation; relative energy deficiency in sport (RED-S), which was previously known as the female athlete triad; and pelvic floor dysfunction.

The Menstrual Cycle and Bone Formation

When an adolescent girl goes through puberty, on average around age thirteen, estrogen increases fat deposition, stimulates breast development, and causes her hips to start to widen. Follicular stimulating hormone (FSH) and luteinizing hormone (LH) are hormones that help eggs to mature and be released. During puberty, these hormones initially surge only at night, which may explain why teen girls need more sleep.[51]

Estrogen plays a vital role in bone health. With missed menstrual cycles, known as amenorrhea, there is decreased estrogen, which leads to decreased bone protection. Ultimately, this causes bones to be broken down, leading to osteopenia and osteoporosis. Please refer to page 164 of the bonus chapter for further discussion.

Relative Energy Deficiency in Sports (RED-S)

Missed periods and decreased bone density lead us into our next topic: relative energy deficiency in sport (RED-S), formerly known as the female athlete triad. This energy-deficient triad includes the following:

1. Low energy availability (usually, but not always, due to an eating disorder)
2. Menstrual dysfunction
3. Low bone mineral density, leading to osteoporosis

It is important to note that RED-S does not just affect adolescents but can be present during later stages during a woman's lifetime. I am mentioning it here because this is the earliest time in a woman's life that it may appear, and catching and addressing it early can help decrease issues later in life. One early sign of RED-S is noticing an absent or abnormal period for three months or greater. If this is the case, your doctor should determine if there are other underlying causes, such as pregnancy, ovarian failure, pituitary tumors, or other issues.

To help reverse effects of RED-S, it is suggested to decrease exercise and training intensity by 10 percent, increase energy intake through nutrition, and/or begin estrogen replacement therapy.[52] This can be a very challenging issue to deal with, especially when an eating disorder is involved. My best advice is to seek out a holistic healthcare approach of counseling, physical therapy, endocrinology, and primary care; other providers may also be able to help.

Pelvic Floor Dysfunction

Just like women in later life stages, adolescent girls can experience pelvic floor dysfunction. As you know well by now, the pelvic floor is just another group of muscles, and issues within these muscles can occur in adolescents. These muscles can be tight and painful or weak, both of which can contribute to bowel and bladder dysfunction. With the start of menstrual cycles, especially if painful, the pelvic floor, low back, and abdominal wall can tense in response. It is important to understand that teenage girls are not excluded from the benefits of pelvic floor physical therapy! There is no need to suffer through this.

REPRODUCTIVE YEARS

Reproductive years begin during puberty with the onset of a woman's menstrual cycle and end at menopause. The three concerns in the adolescence section—importance of a regular menstrual cycle, RED-S, and pelvic floor dysfunction—are also still relevant during the reproductive years of a woman's life. As well, readers should review chapters 8 and 9 for details about pregnancy and postpartum issues.

Of course, the reproductive years extend well beyond the months you may be pregnant or postpartum, and some women will not experience those two stages at all. If you are sexually active, then it is important to have regular gynecology appointments for Pap smear testing, HPV testing, and STD testing. For more information on the details of these tests, please refer to the bonus chapter, "Wellness Screening and Testing."

MENOPAUSE

Similar to puberty, a woman's body goes through many changes as she approaches menopause. Menopause begins one year after a woman's final menstrual period, but she may experience symptoms months to years prior, during the perimenopause period. Estrogen plays a key role in many of the changes noted during this timeframe. A decrease in estrogen production can result in several changes to the pelvic floor, bone health, and mental well-being. What about hot flashes and insomnia?

You guessed it; decreased estrogen levels are usually the culprit. Let's take a closer look.

During menopause, it's important to continue examining your perineum to monitor for changes (see page 26 for detailed instructions). During this time, women can experience vaginal dryness, which can lead to pelvic pain. Estrogen helps to keep vaginal tissue healthy, moisturized, and flexible, and without it, tissue can become dry, thin, and more easily tear. During this time, women are also more prone to experiencing a urethral caruncle, which is pale white, pink, or red dehydrated tissue located around the urethral opening. Sometimes, you won't feel any symptoms, but other times it can bleed or be painful.

It's also extremely important to monitor for vaginal bleeding. Postmenopausal bleeding raises concern for gynecological cancers and needs to be discussed with your doctor immediately. Vulvar cancer, a type of gynecological cancer, is most prevalent in women above fifty years old.[53] A key early detection of this cancer involves noticing changes within the vulvar tissue: sores, rashes, warts, or change in skin color. For more information on gynecologic cancers, refer to page 170 of the bonus chapter.

Due to the decreased estrogen affecting the pelvic floor during the perimenopausal and postmenopausal time frame, physical issues that previously were just small nuisances can now become big problems. If you used to leak just a few drops with sneezing, now you may wet your pants entirely. If you used to just barely make it to the bathroom in time, now you might not make it. If you used to have just a little bit of pain here and there with sex, now you might have more pain more frequently. Maybe you used to feel just a little bit of vaginal pressure but now it has turned into a constant bulging feeling from a pelvic organ prolapse. You get the picture. Still, though, *you should absolutely not accept this as your new "normal."* You have a lot of life left to live, and it's not too late to address any issues you might be having that have been exacerbated during this time. Seek out pelvic floor physical therapy to help.

As we discussed in the adolescence section, estrogen also plays an important role on bone health. During the postmenopausal time frame, there is an increased risk for osteopenia and osteoporosis due to the decreased protective properties on bone from estrogen. For further reading on osteoporosis, please see the next section, "Elderhood," and the bonus chapter, "Wellness Screening and Testing."

Other important topics worth mentioning in this section include depression and heart disease. Symptoms of depression may increase during menopause. This may be due to hormonal fluctuations, but it can also be influenced by potential life changes such as empty nest syndrome and the need to provide care to elderly parents.[54] If you believe you are suffering from depression, please reach out to your health care provider, who can refer you to a counselor, suggest medication, or offer other ways to help.

Did you know your risk of heart disease and heart attacks goes up as you get older? This is also due to a decrease in estrogen. Estrogen helps keep blood vessels relaxed and open, but with decreased estrogen, cholesterol can build up on artery walls, causing thickened and blocked arteries.[55] Please refer to the bonus chapter, "Wellness Screening and Testing," for further information on depression and heart disease.

In general, you should talk to your doctor regarding hormone replacement therapy, diet, and lifestyle modifications to help manage your symptoms during menopause. If you find that your pelvic floor is suffering from any sort of pain, prolapse, bladder issues, or bowel issues, consider seeing a pelvic floor physical therapist!

ELDERHOOD

As you get older and enter elderhood, you will continue to experience changes. It is challenging to define exactly when elderhood begins. Medical doctor and author Louise Aronson informs us that for thousands of years "old" has been defined as beginning between the ages of sixty and seventy. However, she challenges readers to reframe their mind-set on what it means to be an elder. She writes, "We've made old age into a disease, a condition to be dreaded, disparaged, neglected, and denied."[56] Usually, women do not begin feeling that they are "old" or in "elderhood" unless they experience some of the stereotypical issues of mental and physical decline that come with this stage of life,[57] such as arthritis. I believe elderhood should not be viewed as a fearful or dreaded time of life, but rather as a time of continued gratitude and appreciation for life. Let's take a brief look at some of the common challenges that elders experience and how physical therapy can help.

A key change for discussion during elderhood is decreased strength. Sarcopenia is an age-related decrease in muscle mass and decrease in the ability of muscles to regenerate. Even though this is something you cannot change (age is a non-modifiable risk factor), there are measures you can take (modifiable risk factors) to help slow the decline in your loss of strength. These measures include the following:[58]

- Getting adequate nutrition (especially protein)
- Staying as active as possible
- Exercising regularly
- Working with your healthcare providers to properly manage chronic diseases and prevent any new diseases

Ultimately, as you age, sarcopenia will affect your endurance, posture, coordination, and balance. So just what does this mean for your pelvic floor? Similar to during menopause, during elderhood whatever issues you may be experiencing—bladder issues, bowel issues, pelvic organ prolapse, pelvic floor muscle weakness, or pain—will usually become much more problematic.

Do not begin to stress though; pelvic floor physical therapy can still help! By this point in the book, you've learned that there is a huge behavioral component in addressing several of the bladder and bowel issues and that you can see improvement by addressing your behaviors and habits in addition to working on your pelvic floor muscles. Several of my patients are elderly women, and even though their age puts them at a disadvantage for improving pelvic floor muscle strength, they still see positive results. Yes, it can be a little bit harder to change your habits (such as not peeing "just in case"), but this is no reason to throw in the towel. Equally important, maximizing strength of your core and pelvic floor muscles is key to helping decrease your risk of falls, which is a huge concern at this stage of life.

Did you know that women, in particular white women, have the highest incidence of hip fractures? In fact, in the United States, 70 to 75 percent of hip fractures occur in women. After sustaining a hip fracture, the mortality rate increases, and it continues to increase for the ten years that follow the fracture.[59] To make matters more shocking, half of people who sustain a hip fracture will never return to being as active and independent as they were before, and if you are elderly or have other chronic conditions, you are even less likely to regain your independence.[60]

Before you begin to worry about falling, let's talk about what contributes to fall risks and how it can be addressed. During elderhood, fall risk increases not only due to the muscle weakness as a result of sarcopenia, but also because reaction time slows down, which means that if you trip or stumble, you cannot react as quickly to catch yourself. Additionally, your joints lose some of their mobility, resulting in decreased range of motion and increased joint stiffness, which can lead to decreased coordination and, in turn, risk of falling.[61] These aspects are inevitable, so we cannot prevent them from happening. However, you may be thinking that these conditions all sound like areas that physical therapy can help manage—and you are right! A physical therapist can help you take important measures to decrease your risk of falling.

In physical therapy, you will be prescribed a specific program to address your strength, balance, coordination, range of motion, and functional mobility tasks, such as getting in and out of bed, walking, stair climbing, dressing, and so on. You will also be assessed for the appropriate use of an assistive device, such as a walker or a cane, if needed. You will learn home safety, such as removing all tripping hazards like throw rugs and power cords. You will also learn visual scanning techniques to help you look ahead to see where you are going versus only looking down at your feet when walking. The list goes on and on! If you feel you would benefit from physical therapy but are unable to easily make it to the clinic, home physical therapy is available, which means the treatment is done in the comfort of your own home. All you need is for your doctor to specify "home care" when referring you to physical therapy.

The negative effects of menopause on a woman's bones, leading to osteopenia and osteoporosis, are linked to the fact that 70 to 75 percent of people who sustain hip fractures are women. In fact, it is suggested that one in three women over the age of fifty will sustain a fracture related to osteoporosis in her lifetime.[62] For elders, physical therapy can help to manage osteopenia or osteoporosis by prescribing safe, weight-bearing and weight-lifting exercises to help you build your bones.[63] Rest assured, throughout your entire lifespan physical therapists have your back (well, your whole body, really!).

Wellness Screening
and Testing

B Y NOW, I hope you feel confident in navigating the ins-and-outs of
the essential area between your hips. However, because I feel strongly
about preventative care and wellness, I am also including a bonus chapter
to help you determine if and when you need various screening and testing procedures done. Although it's tempting to rely on your healthcare
providers to tell you when you need certain tests done, in reality, we need
to advocate for ourselves. Many providers see upwards of twenty patients
a day, and sadly things get missed. The best approach is to take control
of your health and keep a log (provided Appendix A) of when you've had
testing done. Then you can easily present this log to your doctor to review
and to refer you for any tests required. This bonus chapter covers various
tests a woman may encounter throughout her life.

Please note that the testing and screening information that follows
should serve as general guidelines only; it should not take the place of or
substitute for the testing guidelines suggested by your physician. If you
are concerned about your medical testing and screening, consult your
physician.

BONE MINERAL DENSITY SCAN

A bone mineral density (BMD) scan is an x-ray that looks at the density of your bones (obviously, you gathered that from its name). It is done at your upper thigh bone, low back, wrist bone, or heel bone.

This scan tests for osteoporosis or osteopenia. Osteopenia is bone loss that is not severe enough to yet be classified as osteoporosis. Osteoporosis occurs when bones become fragile from a decrease in density and quality, ultimately causing an increased risk of fractures. You may be at increased risk for osteoporosis if you have one or more of these factors:[64]

- You have a family history of osteoporosis.
- You do not get adequate calcium and vitamin D, which both work to build bone and maintain strong bones.
- You have an eating disorder with menstrual cycle irregularities.
- You have not gotten your period for three months in a row. This may indicate your ovaries are not making enough estrogen, in which case you're also lacking the protective effects it has on bones.
- You are postmenopausal, which results in a decrease in estrogen, which when present helps protect bone density.
- You are a smoker. Smoking causes poor tissue integrity, delayed healing times, and brittle bones with earlier onset of menopause, thus you experience less protective effects of estrogen.
- You are small and thin. There is a law, called Wolff's Law, that states bone is built in response to the stresses that are placed on it. Therefore, with physical activity, a smaller, thinner person generates less stress on their bones, which potentially causes less bone to be built.

With any of these risk factors, your doctor may order a BMD scan. Additionally, if you've experienced more than two stress fractures, you may need a BMD scan. Refer to the "Recommended Resources" section in the back of the book for more information on how to manage osteoporosis and how to quit smoking.

BREAST EXAMS

Get familiar with your breasts! There are three types of breast exams: self, clinical, and imaging.[65]

Self-Breast Exams

Self-breast exams should be performed monthly. It is best to perform the exam a week after your period to avoid tenderness that may come along with your menstrual cycle. If you don't have a period, pick a consistent day of the month that you will remember. I suggest doing your self-breast exam the same day that you take a look at your perineum (discussed on page 26 of chapter 3) to monitor changes. You might as well check all your lady bits at once!

When doing a self-exam, start by standing in front of a mirror and look—yes, check out your boobs! Pay attention to the size, shape, color, any swelling, dimpling, puckering, and other changes in nipple positioning. After you're done looking, lie down and feel each breast, using the tips of your fingers. Use a circular motion from your collar bone moving down to the top of your belly and from your breast bone to your armpit to cover all of the underlying breast tissue, feeling for lumps.

Clinical Breast Exams

These are similar to self-exams, but your doctor performs them during your yearly physical. If you don't see a gynecologist, make sure your primary care physician does this exam for you.

Imaging Exams

These include mammograms and breast MRIs. A mammogram is a low-dose x-ray of the breasts, and an MRI uses magnets and radio waves to take pictures of the breasts. A breast MRI is used for those who are at higher risk for breast cancer. Your healthcare provider will determine whether you need a mammogram or MRI. Women in their forties should begin talking to their healthcare provider about when to start imaging testing. From ages fifty through seventy-four, women will have a mammogram every one to two years depending on their individual risk factors and plan established with their doctor.

COLORECTAL CANCER

You should be screened for colon cancer starting at fifty years old. Screening tests can include the following:[66]

- Stool tests, which look for blood and altered DNA in your poop
- A sigmoidoscopy, which looks at the lower portion of your rectum
- A colonoscopy, which looks at your entire colon
- A CT colonography, which takes an x-ray image of your entire colon

Depending on your medical history and risk factors, your doctor will determine how frequently you need testing and which tests are best for you.

DEPRESSION

Depression is serious. Those of you who have experienced it will know exactly what I mean. There is no "pulling yourself together." You feel trapped, hopeless, and empty. It is more than feeling down or sad. Depression consumes every second of every day, it is always lurking in your mind, and it is always casting its shadow of darkness upon you.

Women are twice as likely to be diagnosed with depression compared to men, but depression is not normal just because you are a woman.[67] Depression presents differently for everybody in regards to what you feel, how long those feelings last, and how severe they are. Some key symptoms of depression include the following:[68]

- Difficulty focusing, decreased memory, and difficulty making decisions
- Feeling easily annoyed, bothered, and angered; feeling moody
- Unrelenting headaches, an upset stomach, and pain

Depression is an illness, just as bronchitis, the flu, and urinary tract infections are all illnesses. Like these other illnesses, there is help for depression, and I encourage you to seek help if you have even an inkling of a suspicion that you may be depressed. Your doctor may prescribe medication and/or counseling to help. Exercise is also encouraged to help release those "feel-good" endorphins.

Let's face it, most women are hard on themselves, and many are afraid to have a stigma placed on them for taking medication. Why is that? Maybe it's because we feel we should be able to manage these feelings on our own. We are tempted to say things like "I'll just do more yoga, practice meditation, work on my relaxation strategies, take up journaling, exercise more" (and so forth). Although these are all great strategies that can certainly help, if you try them and still feel depressed, get professional help! Healthcare providers, including physical therapists, are trained to recognize and screen for signs and symptoms of depression. You can ask your provider to screen you for depression at your next appointment, regardless of what that appointment was originally scheduled for. Otherwise, make an appointment with your primary care physician for further discussion. It can take courage to start this conversation, but ultimately you will find that the results are well worth it. If you are not comfortable pursuing this on your own, please ask a friend or family member to give you the support you need to help you seek professional treatment.

HEART DISEASE

Everyone knows that chest pain and discomfort can be a symptom of a heart attack—but this is mostly true for men.[69] Women usually have a different cluster of signs and symptoms. A woman may experience the following:[70]

- Upper back, neck, jaw, throat, or shoulder pain (usually all left-sided)
- Indigestion
- Heartburn
- A stomachache, nausea, or vomiting
- Extreme fatigue
- Shortness of breath

If you experience any of these symptoms, especially if you are postmeno-pausal, go to the emergency room; it could be a sign of a heart attack.

Cholesterol Levels

A blood test can measure your cholesterol levels, providing insight into your risk for heart disease. Based on your cholesterol levels, your doctor will guide you in dietary and physical activity modifications to help lower your risk of heart disease. A quick review of cholesterol levels include the following:

- Low-density lipopotein (LDL): This is "bad" cholesterol, which leads to a buildup of cholesterol in your arteries.
- High-density lipoprotein (HDL): This is "good" cholesterol, which helps decrease the total cholesterol in your body.
- Total cholesterol: This is LDL and HDL combined, or the total cholesterol in your body.
- Triglycerides: This is a type of fat in your blood that increases your risk for heart disease.

There are no symptoms of high triglyceride levels or high LDL levels; the only way to know is by getting your blood tested. Depending on your medical history and your family history, your doctor will determine the frequency at which you need testing. As a general guideline, it is recommended to have your cholesterol levels checked once prior to puberty between the ages of nine to eleven, once after puberty between the ages of seventeen to twenty-one, and then every four to six years after puberty during adulthood.[71]

Blood Pressure

Like cholesterol, high blood pressure (also known as hypertension) is a contributing factor for heart disease. This is a preventable condition that if undetected or left untreated can lead to heart failure, heart attack, stroke, kidney disease, and death. Ladies, don't be fooled: it is actually just as common in women as it is in men.

You should begin screening for high blood pressure annually, starting at age eighteen.[72] Hypertension is often referred to as "the silent killer" because you usually will not experience any symptoms until it has caused significant damage to your cardiovascular system—all the more reason for regular screening! You are at an increased risk of developing high blood pressure if any of the following conditions apply to you:[73]

- You already experience blood pressure that is slightly elevated: 120/80 to 129/80 mmHg.
- You are diabetic.
- You have an unhealthy diet, especially one that is high in salt.
- You lack regular exercise.
- You are overweight or obese.
- You drink excessive alcohol (for women, that means more than one drink a day).
- You smoke.
- You are older (the risk of high blood pressure increases as we age due to losing elasticity within the blood vessels).
- You are African American.
- You have a family history of high blood pressure.

The good news is that most of these factors are modifiable, which means you can make lifestyle changes to help!

Blood pressure screening is usually done at your doctor's office, but there are home units your doctor may prescribe for you to monitor your blood pressure at home. This is helpful because feeling emotional, stressed, and experiencing pain are factors that can increase your blood pressure reading, and all of these are common factors you may experience when visiting your doctor. Your physical therapist can also monitor your blood pressure during your course of care, so do not hesitate to request this of your physical therapist.

MOLES

Ladies, wear sunscreen and check your skin! I used to be the worst—avoiding sunscreen and even occasionally tanning, striving for that sun-kissed glow. It was not worth it, and I now value my health more than the desire to look "sun-kissed" all year.

It is important to look at your skin and get to know it, just like you should get to know your boobs and vagina! The easiest way to do this is by performing monthly skin checks, which you can do right after you complete your monthly self-breast exam and look at your perineum! As a part of your yearly physical, you can also ask your doctor to check your skin.

When doing your skin check, it's easy as ABCDE—literally:[74]

A = Asymmetry: does one part of the mole not match the other?

B = Border: is the mole edge irregular, ragged, notched, or blurred?

C = Color: are there areas of brown, back, pink, red, white, or blue patches?

D = Diameter: is the mole larger than the size of a pencil eraser?

E = Evolving: is the mole changing over time in size, shape, or color?

If you answered yes to any of these questions, get the mole checked by your doctor.

PAP SMEAR AND HPV TESTING

It's time for your GYN exam, but perhaps you dread your annual appointment. Encountering a cold speculum and having your cervix swabbed likely isn't anyone's favorite thing to do. However, this is a very important test to have done. A Pap smear looks at cervical cells, testing for cervical cancer or cells that look suspicious for becoming cervical cancer. HPV tests are used to detect human papillomavirus, a sexually transmitted infection within your cervix that can lead to cancer or genital warts.

It is suggested that cervical cancer screening should begin at age twenty-one. Women should get tested every three to five years until age sixty-five; your healthcare provider will determine your testing frequency. You no longer need testing if you've had a total hysterectomy with your cervix removed or are over sixty-five years old with a history of normal HPV and Pap testing.[75]

A Pap smear is able to detect cervical cancer only; unfortunately, there are no available screening tests for ovarian, uterine, vaginal, and vulvar cancers. Thus, it is important you are aware of the signs and symptoms for these other gynecological cancers:[76]

Cervical cancer: Abnormal vaginal bleeding or discharge

Ovarian cancer: Abnormal vaginal bleeding or discharge, feeling full too quickly or difficulty eating, feeling bloated, experiencing pelvic pain, abdominal pain, back pain or pelvic pressure, experiencing a more frequent or urgent need to pee, and feeling constipated or bloated

Uterine cancer: Abnormal vaginal bleeding or discharge and experiencing pelvic pain or pressure

Vaginal cancer: Abnormal vaginal bleeding or discharge, experiencing a more frequent or urgent need to pee, and feeling constipated

Vulvar cancer: Experiencing pain, itching, burning or tenderness to the vulva and observing changes within the vulvar tissue: sores, rashes, warts, or change in skin color

As you can see, abnormal vaginal bleeding is a sign of all gynecological cancers except for vulvar cancer, and it is the only sign for cervical cancer. If you experience any abnormal vaginal bleeding, at any age, consult your doctor immediately. This is especially true if you experience postmenopausal bleeding. Examples of abnormal bleeding if you are not postmenopausal include bleeding between periods, heavier than normal periods, and/or periods that last longer than normal.

You may also notice that several of these signs and symptoms look familiar from the issues that have been mentioned throughout this entire book: pelvic pain, pelvic pressure, constipation, and urinary urgency and frequency. This is why it is important to monitor your symptoms and identify what is unique to you. Seek medical attention if you suddenly experience one or more of the warning signs and symptoms associated with gynecological cancer and it lasts more than two weeks.

SEXUALLY TRANSMITTED DISEASES

Sexually transmitted diseases (STDs) or sexually transmitted infections (STIs) may present with symptoms that mimic urinary tract infections or yeast infections, or they may present without symptoms at all. STD testing is different than a Pap smear, which looks for cancerous cells within your cervix. STD testing is done via a pelvic exam, a blood test, a urine test, and/or a vaginal fluid sample.

STD testing is important because if STDs go undetected and untreated, they can cause permanent, serious damage to a woman's reproductive system and lead to chronic pelvic pain.[77] If you are sexually active, discuss your risks with your doctor to determine if and how frequently you should have STD testing. You may feel bashful or embarrassed to begin this conversation, but you don't need to be. The fact is, sex is a normal human desire and a lot of people engage in it. If you don't ask your doctor about STD testing, you put your own health at risk.

The frequency of STD testing depends on your sexual behaviors. You are at a higher risk of having an STD if you meet any of the following criteria:[78]

- Have multiple current sex partners
- Have a new partner
- Do not consistently use condoms
- Have sex while using drugs or alcohol
- Use sex as an exchange for money or drugs

If you engage in any of these high-risk sexual behaviors, at any age, you should ask your doctor to be screened at least annually for STDs such as chlamydia, gonorrhea, HIV, and syphilis. Additionally, if you are sexually active under the age of twenty-five, it is suggested you be screened at least once a year, even if you do not engage in the high-risk sexual behaviors. This reasoning behind this is that younger women will potentially have more new sex partners throughout their lifetime, so they are thought to be at a higher risk for contracting gonorrhea and chlamydia than older women are.[79]

If you are over the age of twenty-five and do not engage in high-risk sexual behavior, then you do not need to be tested annually. In that case, the frequency of testing (if any) will be established by your physician.[80]

A pregnant woman will typically be screened for STDs at her first prenatal visit regardless of sexual risk behavior. This is because STDs during pregnancy, if left untreated, can lead to significant health risks, such as preterm labor and compromised health of the unborn baby.[81]

Closing Remarks

Ladies, I hope you have found this practical guide helpful. Above all else, I hope you feel empowered and encouraged, knowing you are not alone in the journey and struggles you face. I am asking that we as women come together to support and encourage each other. After all, life is better when you sit at a table full of people who lift you up and have your back. I have my patients' back, I have your back, and together, we have each other's back.

Thank you for reading this practical guide. Share it with your friends, practice saying *vagina* ten times out loud and don't be embarrassed by it, and feel liberated understanding what lies between your hips! If you want to continue learning more, check out the Recommended Resources section in Appendix B and follow me on social media:

Instagram: @betweenthehips
Facebook: Between the Hips

And remember, you cannot give from an empty cup. Self-care is the BEST care!

Appendix A: Test-Tracking Log

Name of Test	Date of Test	Testing Location	Person Who Ordered	Results	Follow-Up Care	Date to Retest

Appendix B: Recommended Resources

PELVIC FLOOR PHYSICAL THERAPY DIRECTORIES AND WEBSITES

American Physical Therapy Association (APTA). The Academy of Pelvic Health Physical Therapy section of the APTA is "a community of physical therapy professionals changing the conversation and perception about pelvic and abdominal health issues worldwide." You can use their site to locate a pelvic floor physical therapist near you.
ptl.womenshealthapta.org

Herman and Wallace Pelvic Rehabilitation Institute. This site was created "so that patients can easily search the thousands of clinicians that [the institute] trains[s] each year to find the provider that best meets their needs."
pelvicrehab.com

Intimate Rose. Amanda Olson, DPT, PRPC, created this site because she loves "to work with women to support, guide, and cheer them on towards reaching their personal goals." You can also use this website to find a provider.
www.intimaterose.com/pages/find-a-providers

Maven Clinic. Maven Clinic is a women and family telemedicine network that provides telemedicine not only for physical therapy but also for health needs related to preconception, breastfeeding, pregnancy, fertility, adoption, and more.
www.mavenclinic.com

Pelvic Guru. As noted on the website, "The mission of Pelvic Guru is to provide information about pelvic health to a global community in order to improve access to skilled healthcare providers, education, and online resources while normalizing conversations and reducing shame and embarrassment for those who live with their own pelvic health issues." The directory can help you find a provider near you.
www.pelvicguru.com/directory

BREASTFEEDING, REPRODUCTION, AND MOTHERHOOD PODCASTS, BOOKS, AND WEBSITES

The Badass Breastfeeding Podcast. This podcast addresses issues surrounding breastfeeding and motherhood. Host Dianne Cassidy is an International Board-Certified Lactation Consultant, Certified Child Birth Educator, and registered nurse. Host Abby Theuring is a mother who experienced her own breastfeeding struggles and was motivated to do something about it to help other women through their struggles. Visit their website for podcast information and resources on how to find a lactation consultant, breastfeeding book recommendations, and information on other topics such as sex, sleep, childbirth, and nursing. badassbreastfeedingpodcast.com

Birthfit. This podcast (and program) is designed to promote awareness and enhance education throughout the motherhood transition. Founder Dr. Lindsey Mathews, DC, is a doctor of chiropractic, birth doula, strength and conditioning coach, and NLP practitioner who is dedicated to supporting and educating all people throughout the motherhood transition. The podcast is geared toward women during all stages of their journey to motherhood. Visit this website for blog posts, webinars, recommended books for pregnancy and beyond, online exercise programs, and more information on coaching. www.birthfit.com

The Boob Group. This podcast helps new breastfeeding moms maximize their success and provides helpful tips to seasoned moms who are new listeners. It specifically discusses breastfeeding tips during each stage of your baby's life, beginning from the first twenty-four hours! www.theboobgroup.libsyn.com

Breastfeeding Mommas. Raquel, a mom who struggled with breastfeeding herself, founded this useful website to share breastfeeding tips to boost your milk supply, tips to overcome breastfeeding challenges, and breastfeeding product reviews. www.breastfeedingmommas.com

The First Latch. This podcast is hosted by Barbara Demske, who is a mom, nurse, and International Board-Certified Lactation Consultant. The mission of this podcast is to create a nonjudgmental platform to help support and encourage women through their breastfeeding journey no matter what it looks like. Moms and healthcare professionals are interviewed to share their expertise and stories on motherhood and breastfeeding. Visit the website for information on podcast episodes, breastfeeding tips, and mom and baby product reviews. www.thefirstlatch.net

Lactation Link. This website offers webinars, classes, and consultations for breastfeeding moms. Lindsey Shipley, the founder, is a nurse, Childbirth Educator, International Board-Certified Lactation Consultant, Certified Lactation Coach, and mom who observed breastfeeding struggles with her patients and wanted to make information more readily available. Through this link, you can access a free breastfeeding breakthrough course to learn how to get the best latch, decrease problems and pain, and improve breastfeeding efficiency. www.lactationlink.com

San Diego Breastfeeding Center, LLC. This website includes information on virtual and in-person breastfeeding consultations, classes, and support groups; online educational material; and blog posts. Blog posts include categories of baby sleep and feeding cycles from three months to one year and breastfeeding videos—just to name a few! www.sdbfc.com

Taking Charge of Your Fertility: The Definitive Guide to Natural Birth Control, Pregnancy Achievement, and Reproductive Healthy by Toni Weschler, MPH (William Morrow, 2015). In this book, author and women's health educator Toni Weschler provides a plethora of knowledge about a woman's menstrual cycle and fertility signs to assist with avoiding or achieving pregnancy. She explains the Fertility Awareness Method and provides detailed illustrations and graphs to assist you in this journey. www.tcoyf.com

DOMESTIC VIOLENCE HOTLINES AND WEBSITES

National Domestic Violence Hotline. If you are a victim of domestic violence, please seek help by calling the National Domestic Violence Hotline, which is open 24/7, at 800-799-SAFE (7233). You can also talk with one of their advocates by visiting their website.
www.thehotline.org

Office on Women's Health (OWH). The mission of OWH is to "provide national leadership and coordination to improve the health of women and girls through policy, education, and innovative programs." You can call the OWH HELPLINE at 1-800-994-9662 between 9 a.m. and 6 p.m. ET, Monday through Friday. Their website also provides information on domestic violence.
www.womenshealth.gov/relationships-and-safety/domestic-violence

DRUG AND ALCOHOL ABUSE HOTLINES AND WEBSITES

Alcoholics Anonymous (AA). This "nonprofessional, self-supporting, and apolitical" nonprofit organization helps people of all ages and backgrounds with their drinking problem. Visit their website to learn more about Alcoholics Anonymous and other resources, to find a group near you, and to read daily reflections on overcoming alcoholism.
www.aa.org

American Addiction Centers. This website offers access to hotlines for cocaine, heroin, marijuana, meth, and/or opiate abuse and addiction; you can also use it to find a substance abuse resource center near you.
www.drugabuse.com/addiction/drug-abuse-hotlines

National Institute on Alcohol Abuse and Alcoholism (NIAAA). NIAAA is a research-based organization that provides education on the effects of alcohol on health; information on research studies; educational material; and an alcohol treatment navigator to find alcohol programs, therapists, and doctors near you.
www.niaaa.nih.gov

Substance Abuse and Mental Health Services Administration (SAMHSA). SAMHSA's mission is "to reduce the impact of substance use and mental illness on America's communities." Their website can help you find treatment facilities confidentially and anonymously.
www.samhsa.gov

FALL PREVENTION WEBSITES

Centers for Disease Control and Prevention (CDC). The CDC's website offers useful facts and tips on fall prevention.
www.cdc.gov/homeandrecreationalsafety/falls/adultfalls.html

National Council on Aging (NCOA). The NCOA website is dedicated to "keeping older adults safe and active." They offer links to help you find proven programs to prevent falls.
www.ncoa.org/healthy-aging/falls-prevention

MENTAL HEALTH HOTLINES, WEBSITES, PODCASTS, AND BOOKS

National Suicide Prevention Hotline. As the website notes, "We can all help prevent suicide. The Lifeline provides 24/7, free and confidential support for people in distress, prevention and crisis resources for you or your loved ones, and best practices for professionals." Please call 911 or the National Suicide Prevention Lifeline at 1-800-273-TALK (8255) if you are thinking about hurting or killing yourself.
www.suicidepreventionlifeline.org

Substance Abuse and Mental Health Services Administration (SAMHSA). SAMHSA's mission is "to reduce the impact of substance use and mental illness on America's communities." Their website can help you find behavioral healthcare providers near you.
www.samhsa.gov

The Brendon Show. In this podcast, Brendon Burchard, a high-performance coach, shares his strategies and provokes deeper thought on how to lead an extraordinary life. He is also the author of *High Performance Habits: How Extraordinary People Become That Way* (Hay House, 2017).
www.highperformanceinstitute.com

The Happiness Lab. Laurie Santos, who teaches Yale's most popular class, "The Science of Well-Being," leads this podcast. Visit the website to listen and to sign up for newsletters.
www.happinesslab.fm

The Minimalist. This podcast will help you discover that happiness can be found through life itself versus material goods. Visit the website to listen, access related resources, and to sign up for newsletters.
www.theminimalists.com

Celebrate Muliebrity. Visit pelvic health physical therapist Michelle Lyon's website for blog posts on celebrating muliebrity, meaning womanhood.
www.celebratemuliebrity.com

The Body Keeps the Score: Brain, Mind, and Body in the Healing of Trauma by Bessel van der Kolk, MD (Penguin, 2015). In this book, trauma expert Dr. van der Kolk sheds light on holistic strategies of addressing the brain, mind, and body to heal trauma. He provides insight on how past experiences, especially traumatic ones, can affect the body, even years later.

Do One Thing Every Day That Makes You Happy: A Journal (Do One Thing Every Day Journals) by Robie Rogge and Dian G. Smith (Clarkson Potter, 2017). This journal provides daily prompts and mental exercises for self-reflection on what truly makes you happy. It facilitates gratitude and helps you discover the simple encounters that aid in your overall happiness.

Girl, Wash Your Face and *Girl, Stop Apologizing* by Rachel Hollis (Thomas Nelson, 2019). In this two-book set, entrepreneur and life and business coach Rachel Hollis empowers readers by providing strategies to make permanent and lasting positive change in their lives.

Whatever You Are Be a Good One: 100 Inspirational Quotations Hand-Lettered by Lisa Congdon (Chronicle Books, 2014). This book can help brighten your day by providing inspiration, provoking thought, and reminding you to cherish each moment of each day.

Wherever You Go, There You Are: Mindfulness Meditation in Everyday Life by Jon Kabat-Zinn, Ph.D (Hachette, 2005). In this book, scientist, writer, meditation teacher, and author Jon Kabat-Zinn discusses the power and benefits of mindfulness to aid in consciously experiencing life to the fullest potential.

Wolfpack: How to Come Together, Unleash Our Power and Change the Game by Abby Wambach (Celadon, 2019). Abby Wambach is an author, two-time Olympic gold medalist, and FIFA World Cup champion who calls for women to unite and empower each other. She writes about the idea of a wolfpack, where women band together, to create positive change in the world.

A Woman's Book of Inspiration: Quotes of Wisdom and Strength by Carol Kelly-Gangi, ed. (Fall River Press, 2017). This book is filled with quotes from women of all backgrounds and eras, sharing the struggles they faced, providing you with encouragement and inspiration.

OSTEOPOROSIS WEBSITES AND BOOKS

National Osteoporosis Foundation. This foundation is "committed to preventing osteoporosis and promoting awareness about bone health." Check out this website to learn more about bone health basics, prevention and healthy living, nutrition, and safe exercises to help you stay healthy.
www.nof.org

Office on Women's Health (OWH). You can call the OWH hotline for resources from 9 a.m. to 6 p.m. ET, Monday through Friday, at 1-800-994-9662. Their website also provides answers to many common questions about osteoporosis.
www.womenshealth.gov/a-z-topics/osteoporosis

Exercise for Better Bones: The Complete Guide to Safe and Effective Exercises for Osteoporosis, 3rd Edition by Margaret Martin (Kamajojo Press, 2015). In this guide the author, who is a physical therapist and certified strength and conditioning coach, provides evidence-based exercise programs from the beginner level to the elite level to build bone density for those with osteoporosis, osteopenia, or low bone density. You can also download an exercise plan associated with the material. www.melioguide.com/exercise-plans

SEXUAL ASSAULT HOTLINES AND WEBSITES

National Sexual Assault Hotline. If you are a victim of sexual assault, call the hotline at 800-656-HOPE (4673) to connect with a sexual assault service provider in your area who can direct you to local resources. If you are in the military, you may also call the *Department of Defense Safe Helpline* at 877-995-5247.

Office on Women's Health (OWH). If you have been sexually assaulted or raped, visit their website to learn about the appropriate steps to get help and medical attention.
www.womenshealth.gov/relationships-and-safety/sexual-assault-and-rape/sexual-assault

SMOKING HOTLINES AND WEBSITES

Centers for Disease Control and Prevention (CDC). The CDC's website offers tips and support to help you quit smoking.
www.cdc.gov/tobacco/campaign/tips

U.S. Department of Health and Human Services. For help to quit smoking and to learn of support services in your area, call 1-800-QUIT-NOW (1-800-784-8669). You can also visit their website for articles, tools, and tips.
www.smokefree.gov

PELVIC PAIN AND WELLNESS BOOKS, PODCASTS, AND WEBSITES

Beating Endo: How to Reclaim Your Life from Endometriosis by Iris Kerin Orbuch, MD and Amy Stein, DPT (Harper Wave, 2019). In this book, you will learn how to use a holistic approach to manage and conquer your fight with endometriosis, which often coincides with pelvic floor muscle, bladder, and bowel dysfunction. Topics include physical therapy, nutrition, mindfulness, and situational considerations to help overcome endometriosis.

GUT: The Inside Story of Our Body's Most Underrated Organ by Giulia Enders, MD (Greystone Books, 2018). In this book Dr. Enders creatively and cleverly unveils the fascinating science behind our gut. She uses easy-to-understand illustrations and covers the complex integrations between gut health and topics like mental health and autoimmune diseases.

*A Headache in the Pelvis: A New Understanding and Treatment for Chronic Pelvic Pain Syndrome*s by David Wise, Ph.D. and Rodney Anderson, MD (Harmony, 2018). This book discusses Dr. David Wise's twenty-year history of pelvic pain and the approach that he, along with Dr. Anderson, a urologist, utilized to resolve it. This book emphasizes the importance of using a holistic treatment approach of physical therapy, meditation, relaxation strategies, and the behavioral and psychological components behind your pain.

Heal Pelvic Pain: The Proven Stretching, Strengthening, and Nutrition Program for Relieving Pain, Incontinence, I.B.S., and Other Symptoms Without Surgery by Amy Stein, M.P.T. (McGraw-Hill, 2008). In this book, physical therapist Amy Stein addresses pelvic pain by teaching readers about exercise, nutrition, massage, and self-care strategies to address the underlying cause of their pain.

The V-Hive. This podcast is founded and hosted by Hannah Matluck, who suffered herself with years of pelvic pain. In this podcast, Hannah interviews top medical experts on any and every women's intimate health topic.
www.thevhive.com

Intimate Rose. Visit pelvic health physical therapist Amanda Olson's website Intimate Rose to read about success stories; for information on how to use pelvic floor muscle wands, dilators, and vaginal weights; and to read blog posts on all things pelvic health.
www.intimaterose.com

Ohnut. The mission of this company is to help women who struggle with painful sex. The "Ohnut" is a device that is designed to decrease deep pelvic pain with penetrative intercourse. In addition to buying products, you can also sign up for newsletters to learn the latest research and to find support in knowing you are not alone in your journey to eliminate pelvic pain.
www.ohnut.co

Office on Women's Health (OWH). The mission of OWH is to "provide national leadership and coordination to improve the health of women and girls through policy, education, and innovative programs." You can call the OWH HELPLINE at 1-800-994-9662 between 9 a.m. and 6 p.m. ET, Monday through Friday. Their website covers a wide range of topics on women's health.
www.womenshealth.gov/a-z-topics

PREGNANCY LOSS, TRAUMATIC BIRTH, SURROGACY, AND ADOPTION WEBSITES

American Adoptions. This is a not-for-profit domestic adoption agency that works with people looking to place their child with a new family and people looking to adopt a child. This organization works with children ranging in age from newborns to teenagers. Their website includes articles about navigating related emotions, provides 24/7 counseling support, offers women and families a chance to talk to an adoption

specialist, and much more.
www.americanadoptions.com

The Compassionate Friends. This organization offers in-person and virtual support groups for anyone experiencing the loss of a child—no matter age or cause. Visit their website to find a support group near you, enroll in virtual support groups, read blog posts, and view book recommendations.
www.compassionatefriends.org

March of Dimes. This organization focuses on pregnancy health for both mom and baby and advocates for research on preventing birth defects and infant death. Visit their website to learn about the in-person and online options for prenatal and NICU education and support in addition to various resources for the pregnancy and postpartum time-frame—including complications and loss.
www.marchofdimes.org

MISS Foundation. This organization provides C.A.R.E. services (Counseling, Advocacy, Research, and Education) to those who have experienced the loss of a child at any age. Visit their website to learn how to access their services.
www.missfoundation.org

Prevention and Treatment of Traumatic Childbirth (PATTCh). PATTCh's mission is to "expand awareness and advance knowledge about traumatic birth and its adverse impact on all childbearing people and babies." Visit their website to access online learning, articles and blog posts, and support groups on traumatic birth experiences.
www.pattch.org

Share Pregnancy and Infant Loss Support. This is a community of support for anyone who has experienced the loss of a baby through pregnancy loss, stillbirth, or during the first few months of life. This group also provides supports for healthcare professionals who provide care for grieving families. Visit their website to learn about the abundant support resources offered—phone support, in-person support groups, and

online brochures on strategies to manage grief and loss.
www.nationalshare.org

Solace for Mothers. This organization's mission is "to create support for individuals who have been traumatized by the childbearing experiences." They provide online forums and resources for women and families to connect with others who have experienced traumatic childbirth, and they provide a directory of mental health providers who specialize in this topic.
www.solaceformothers.org

Still Standing Magazine, LLC. This resource aims to provide "an online voice in breaking the silence on child loss—from conception to adulthood, and infertility." If you have experienced or struggled with these challenges, visit their website to join an online support group and to read or subscribe to posted articles.
www.stillstandingmag.com

Surrogate.com. This website provides information for surrogates and intended parents on the surrogacy process. It also includes a blog post that provides surrogacy support resources for virtual support groups and further online resources.
www.surrogate.com/surrogates/people-involved-in-your-surrogacy/7-surrogacy-support-resources-for-prospective-surrogates

Notes

1. The Great Wall of Vagina, Jamie McCartney, www.greatwallofvagina.co.uk/home.

2. W. Jerod Greer, Holly E. Richter, Alfred A. Bartolucci, and Kathryn L. Burgio, "Obesity and Pelvic Floor Disorders: A Systematic Review," *Obstetrics & Gynecology* 112, no. 2 Pt 1 (August 2008): 6, doi: 10.1097/AOG.0b013e31817cfdde.

3. Ingeborg Hoff Braekken, Memona Majida, Marie Ellstrom Engh, and Kari Bo, "Can Pelvic Floor Muscle Training Reverse Pelvic Organ Prolapse and Reduce Prolapse Symptoms? An Assessor-Blinded, Randomized, Controlled Trial," *American Journal of Obstetrics & Gynecology* 203, no. 2 (August 2010): 170e4-170e6, doi: doi.org/10.1016/j.ajog.2010.02.037; Suzanne Hagen and Diane Stark, "Conservative Prevention and Management of Pelvic Organ Prolapse in Women (Review)," *Cochrane Database of Systematic Reviews* 12, no. CD003882 (December 2011): 13–14, doi: 10.1002/14651858.CD003882.pub4.

4. Diana T. Sanchez, Amy K. Kiefer, and Oscar Ybarra, "Sexual Submissiveness in Women: Costs for Sexual Autonomy and Arousal," *Personality and Social Psychology Bulletin* 32, no. 4 (April 2006): 512–522, doi: 10.1177/0146167205282154; Osomo Kontula and Anneli Miettinen, "Determinants of Female Sexual Orgasm," *Socioaffective Neuroscience & Psychology* 6, no. 31624 (October 2016): 18–20, doi: 10.3402/snp.v6.31624.

5. Kontula and Miettinen, "Determinants of Female Sexual Orgasm," 1–2.

6. Charlene L. Muehlenhard and Sheena K. Shippee, "Men's and Women's Reports of Pretending Orgasm," *Journal of Sex Research* 47, no. 6 (November 2010): 552, doi: 10.1080/00224490903171794.

7. Debby Herbenick, Tsung-Chieh Jane Fu, Jennifer Arter, Stephanie A. Sanders, and Brian Dodge, "Women's Experiences With Genital Touching, Sexual Pleasure, and Orgasm: Results From a U.S. Probability Sample of Women Ages 18 to 94," *Journal of Sex and Marital Therapy* 44, no. 2 (February 2018): 201, doi: 10.1080/0092623X.2017.1346530; Kontula and Miettinen, "Determinants of Female Sexual Orgasm," 10.

8. Vincenzo Puppo, "Embryology and Anatomy of the Vulva: The Female Orgasm and Women's Sexual Health," *European Journal of Obstetrics & Gynecology and Reproductive Biology* 154, no. 1 (January 2011): 4, doi: doi.

org/10.1016/j.ejogrb.2010.08.009.

9. Amichai Kilchevsky, Yoram Vardi, Lior Lowenstein, and Ilan Gruenwald, "Is the Female G-Spot Truly a Distinct Anatomic Entity?" *Journal of Sexual Medicine* 9, no. 3 (March 2012): 719, doi: 10.1111/j.1743-6109.2011.02623.x.

10. Randi M. Cohen, dir. *Explained: The Female Orgasm*, Vox Media, 2018. www.netflix.com/title/80216752.

11. Good Clean Love, Wendy Strgar, www.goodcleanlove.com.

12. Toni Weschler, *Taking Charge of Your Fertility: The Definitive Guide to Natural Birth Control, Pregnancy Achievement, and Reproductive Health*, 20th Anniversary Edition (New York: William Morrow Paperbacks, 2015).

13. Anna Adams, "Menstrual Cup Misuse 'Can Cause Pelvic Organ Prolapse,'" BBC News, March 11, 2020, www.bbc.com/news/health-51805689.

14. FLEX, www.flexfits.com.

15. Raul Raz, Bibiana Chazan, and Michael Dan, "Cranberry Juice and Urinary Tract Infection," *Clinical Infectious Disease* 38, no. 10 (May 2004): 1414, doi: 10.1086/386328.

16. Prelief, www.prelief.com.

17. Giulia Enders, *Gut: The Inside Story of Our Body's Most Underrated Organ* (Vancouver: Greystone Books, 2015).

18. Brian E. Lacy, Fermin Mearin, Lin Chang, William D. Chey, Anthony J. Lembo, Magnus Simren, and Robin Spiller, "Bowel Disorders," *Gastroenterology* 150, no. 6 (May 2016): 1394, 1399, doi: doi.org/10.1053/j.gastro.2016.02.031.

19. American Psychiatric Association, "Diagnostic and Statistical Manual of Mental Disorders," in *Highlights of Change from DSM-IV-TR to DSM-5,* 5th Edition (Washington DC: American Psychiatric Publishing, 2013).

20. G. Peter Herbison and Nicola Dean, "Weighted Vaginal Cones for Urinary Incontinence," *Cochrane Database of Systematic Reviews* 7, no. CD002114 (July 2013): 12, doi: 10.1002/14651858.CD002114.pub2.

21. Annelie Gutke, Ann Josefsson, and Birgitta Oberg, "Pelvic Girdle Pain and Lumbar Pain in Relation to Postpartum Depressive Symptoms," *Spine* 32, no. 13 (June 2007): 1432–1433, doi: 10.1097/BRS.0b013e318060a673.

22. Erin E. Butler, Iris Colon, Maurice L. Druzin, and Jessica Rose, "Postural Equilibrium During Pregnancy: Decreased Stability With an Increased Reliance on Visual Cues," *American Journal of Obstetrics and Gynecology* 195, no. 4 (October 2006): 1105–1107, doi: 10.1016/j.ajog.2006.06.015.

23. Jean M. Irion and Glenn L. Irion, "Physiological, Anatomical, and

Musculoskeletal Changes during the Childbearing Years," in *Women's Health in Physical Therapy*, edited by Jean M. Irion and Glenn L. Irion (Philadelphia: Lippincott Williams & Wilkins, 2010), 209.

24. Irion and Irion, "Physiological, Anatomical, and Musculoskeletal Changes during the Childbearing Years," 213.

25. Diane G. Lee, "*The Pelvic Girdle: An Integration of Clinical Expertise and Research, Fourth Edition* (London: Churchill Livingstone, 2011), 134.

26. Irion and Irion, "Physiological, Anatomical, and Musculoskeletal Changes during the Childbearing Years," 219–220.

27. Irion and Irion, "Physiological, Anatomical, and Musculoskeletal Changes during the Childbearing Years," 212, 220.

28. Irion and Irion, "Physiological, Anatomical, and Musculoskeletal Changes during the Childbearing Years," 212–213.

29. Irion and Irion, "Physiological, Anatomical, and Musculoskeletal Changes during the Childbearing Years," 215–217.

30. Irion and Irion, "Physiological, Anatomical, and Musculoskeletal Changes during the Childbearing Years," 214.

31. Joanne Borg-Stein and Sheila A. Dugan, "Musculoskeletal Disorders of Pregnancy, Delivery, and Postpartum," *Physical Medicine and Rehabilitation Clinics of North America* 18, no. 3 (August 2007): 460, doi: 10.1016/j.pmr.2007.05.005.

32. Catherine Cram, "Physical Activity and Exercise During the Childbearing Years," in *Women's Health in Physical Therapy*, edited by Jean M. Irion and Glenn L. Irion (Philadelphia: Lippincott Williams & Wilkins, 2010), 254.

33. Special Communications: Roundtable Consensus Statement, "Impact of Physical Activity During Pregnancy and Postpartum on Chronic Disease Risk," *Medicine and Science in Sports and Exercise* 38, no. 5 (May 2006): 990, 1001 doi: 10.1249/01.mss.0000218147.51025.8a.

34. Committee on Obstetric Practice with Meredith L. Birsner and Cynthia Gyamfi-Bannerman, "Physical Activity and Exercise During Pregnancy and the Postpartum Period: ACOG Committee Opinion Summary, Number 804," *Obstetrics & Gynecology* 135, no. 4 (April 2020), doi: 10.1097/AOG.0000000000003773.

35. Jean M. Irion and Glenn L. Irion, "Physical Therapy Interventions During Labor and Delivery and Postpartum Care," in *Women's Health in Physical Therapy*, edited by Jean M. Irion and Glenn L. Irion (Philadelphia: Lippincott

Williams & Wilkins, 2010), 309; John Dame, Jon Neher, and Sarah Safranek, "Clinical Inquiries: Does Antepartum Perineal Massage Reduce Intrapartum Laceration?" *The Journal of Family Practice* 57, no. 7 (July 2008): 480–481, PMID: 18625174.

36. Jean M. Irion and Glenn L. Irion, "Medical Management and Physical Therapy Management of High-Risk Pregnancy," in *Women's Health in Physical Therapy*, edited by Jean M. Irion and Glenn L. Irion (Philadelphia: Lippincott Williams & Wilkins, 2010), 328–351.

37. Jill S. Boissonnault, William G. Boissonnault, and Patricia Bartoli, "Osteoporosis During the Childbearing Year," *Journal of Women's Health Physical Therapy* 29, no. 3 (December 2005): 28, 31, journals.lww.com/jwhpt/toc/2005/29030.

38. Irion and Irion, "Physical Therapy Interventions During Labor and Delivery and Postpartum Care," 295–296.

39. Jing Huang, Yu Zang, Li-Hau Ren, Feng-Juan Li, and Hong Lu, "A Review and Comparison of Common Maternal Positions During the Second-Stage of Labor," *International Journal of Nursing Sciences* 6, no. 4 (October 2019): 464, doi: doi.org/10.1016/j.ijnss.2019.06.007.

40. Jing Huang, Yu Zang, Li-Hau Ren, Feng-Juan Li, and Hong Lu, "A Review and Comparison," 463.

41. Janesh K. Gupta, Akanksha Sood, G. Justus Hofmeyr, and Joshua P. Vogel, "Position in the Second Stage of Labour for Women Without an Epidural Anaesthesia," *Cochrane Database of Systematic Reviews* 5, no. CD002006 (May 2017): 2, doi: 10.1002/14651858.CD002006.pub4.

42. "Can Vaginal Seeding After a C-Section Benefit My Baby?" Mayo Clinic, last modified October 04, 2019, www.mayoclinic.org/healthy-lifestyle/infant-and-toddler-health/expert-answers/vaginal-seeding/faq-20380881; Committee on Obstetric Practice with Kurt R. Wharton and Meredith L. Birsner, "Vaginal Seeding: ACOG Committee Opinion, Number 725," *Obstetrics & Gynecology* 130, no. 5 (November 2017): e274, doi: 10.1097/AOG.0000000000002402; Giulia Enders, *Gut: The Inside Story of Our Body's Most Underrated Organ* (Vancouver: Greystone Books, 2015), 165–166.

43. Committee on Obstetric Practice with Maria A. Mascola, T. Flint Porter, and Tamara Tin-May Chao, "Delayed Umbilical Cord Clamping After Birth: ACOG Committee Opinion, Number 684," *Obstetrics & Gynecology* 129, no. 1 (January 2017): e5, doi: 10.1097/AOG.0000000000001860.

44. Amy R. Palmer and Frances E. Likis, "Lactational Atrophic Vaginitis," *Journal of Midwifery & Women's Health* 48, no.4 (December 2010): 282–284, doi: doi.org/10.1016/S1526-9523(03)00143-0.

45. Cram, "Physical Activity and Exercise During the Childbearing Years," 265.

46. Special Communications: Roundtable Consensus Statement, "Impact of Physical Activity During Pregnancy and Postpartum on Chronic Disease Risk," *Medicine and Science in Sports and Exercise* 38, no. 5 (May 2006): 997–998, doi: 10.1249/01.mss.0000218147.51025.8a.

47. Jean Y. Ko, Karilynn M. Rockhill, Van T. Tong, Brian Morrow, and Sherry L. Farr, "Trends in Postpartum Depressive Symptoms – 27 States, 2004, 2008, and 2012," *Morbidity and Mortality Weekly Report* 66, no. 6 (February 2017): 157, doi: 10.15585/mmwr.mm6606a1.

48. The American College of Obstetricians and Gynecologists. "Postpartum Depression: Frequently Asked Questions Labor, Delivery, and Postpartum Care," FAQ091, 2019, www.acog.org/patient-resources/faqs/labor-delivery-and-postpartum-care/postpartum-depression.

49. Rachel Hollis, *Girl, Wash Your Face: Stop Believing the Lies About Who You Are So You Can Become Who You Were Meant to Be* (Nashville: Thomas Nelson, 2018).

50. I.E. Nygaard, F.L. Thompson, S.L. Svengalis, and J.P. Albright, "Urinary Incontinence in Elite Nulliparous Athletes," *Obstetrics and Gynecology* 84, no. 2 (August 1994): abstract, PMID: 8041527.

51. Jessica R. Drummond, "The Adolescent Female," in *Women's Health in Physical Therapy,* edited by Jean M. Irion and Glenn L. Irion (Philadelphia: Lippincott Williams & Wilkins, 2010), 364.

52. Karen Birch, "*ABC of Sports and Exercise Medicine:* Female Athlete Triad," *The BMJ* 330, no. 7485 (January 2005): 246, doi: 10.1136/bmj.330.7485.244.

53. "Risk Factors for Vulvar Cancer," Cancer Treatment Centers of America, www.cancercenter.com/cancer-types/vulvar-cancer/risk-factors.

54. David A. Kahn, Margaret L. Moline, Ruth W. Ross, Lori L. Altshuler, and Lee S. Cohen, "Depression During the Transition to Menopause: A Guide for Patients and Families," *Postgraduate Medical Journal* Spec No: 114–115 (March 2001): 2, PMID: 11501001.

55. "Menopause and Heart Disease," American Heart Association, last modified July 31, 2015, www.heart.org/en/health-topics/consumer-healthcare/what-is-cardiovascular-disease/menopause-and-heart-disease.

56. "Elderhood," Louis Aronson, www.louisearonson.com/books/elderhood.

57. Louis Aronson, *Elderhood: Redefining Aging, Transforming Medicine, Reimagining Life* (London: Bloomsbury Publishing, 2019).

58. Susan B. O'Sullivan, Thomas J. Schmitz, and George D. Fulk, "Examination of Coordination and Balance," in *Physical Rehabilitation Seventh Edition,* ed. Edward W. Bezkor and Evangelos Pappas (Philadelphia: F.A. Davis Compay, 2019), 197.

59. Robert S. Sterling, "Gender and Race/Ethnicity Differences in Hip Fractures Incidence, Morbidity, Mortality, and Function," *Clinical Orthopaedics Related Research* 469, no. 7 (July 2011): 1913, 1915, doi: 10.1007/s11999-010-1736-3.

60. Victoria L. Tang, Rebecca Sudore, Irena Stijacic Cenzer, W. John Boscardin, Alex Smith, Christine Ritchie, Margaret Wallhagen, Emily Finlayson, Laura Petrillo, and Kenneth Covinsky, "Rates of Recovery to Pre-Fracture Function in Older Persons with Hip Fracture: an Observational Study," *Journal of General Internal Medicine* 32, no.3 (September 2016): 156, doi: 10.1007/s11606-016-3848-2.

61. O'Sullivan, Schmitz, and Fulk, "Examination of Coordination and Balance," 197–198.

62. Tumay Sozen, Lale Ozisik and Nursel Calik Basaran, "An Overview and Management of Osteoporosis," *European Journal of Rheumatology* 4, no. 1 (March 2017): 46, doi: 10.5152/eurjrheum.2016.048.

63. Carol Hamilton Zehnacker and Anita Bemis-Dougherty, "Effect of Weighted Exercises on Bone Mineral Density in Post Menopausal Women: A Systematic Review," *Journal of Geriatric Physical Therapy* 30, no. 2 (August 2007): 87, doi: 10.1519/00139143-200708000-00007.

64. Elizabeth A. Joy, Sonja Van Hala, and Leslie Cooper, "Health-Related Concerns of the Female Athlete: A Lifespan Approach," *American Family Physician* 79, no. 6 (March 2009): 493, PMID: 19323362; "Osteoporosis," Office on Women's Health, last modified May 20, 2019, www.womenshealth.gov/a-z-topics/osteoporosis.

65. "Breast Self-Exam," BreastCancer.Org, last modified October 24, 2019, www.breastcancer.org/symptoms/testing/types/self_exam; "What Is Breast Cancer Screening?" Centers for Disease Control and Prevention, last modified September 11, 2018, www.cdc.gov/cancer/breast/basic_info/screening.htm.

66. "Colorectal Cancer Screening Tests," Centers for Disease Control and

Prevention, last modified February 10, 2020, www.cdc.gov/cancer/colorectal/
basic_info/screening/tests.htm.

67. Paul R. Albert, "Why is Depression More Prevalent in Women?" *Journal of
Psychiatry & Neuroscience* 40, no. 4 (July 2105): 219, doi: 10.1503/jpn.150205.

68. "Depression," Office on Women's Health, last modified May 14, 2019,
www.womenshealth.gov/mental-health/mental-health-conditions/depression.

69. John G. Canto, William J. Rogers, Robert J. Goldberg, Eric D. Peterson,
Nanette K. Wenger, Viola Vaccarino, Catarina I. Kiefe, Paul D. Frederick,
George Sopko, and Zhi-Jie Zheng, "Association of Age and Sex With Myo-
cardial Infarction Symptom Presentation and In-Hospital Mortality," *Journal
of the American Medical Association* 307, no. 8 (July 2015): 2, doi: 10.1001/
jama.2012.199.

70. Glenn Irion, "Women and Heart Disease," in *Women's Health in Physical
Therapy,* edited by Jean M. Irion and Glenn L. Irion (Philadelphia: Lippincott
Williams & Wilkins, 2010), 461.

71. "How and When to Have Your Cholesterol Checked," Centers for Disease
Control and Prevention, last modified September 7, 2018, www.cdc.gov/fea-
tures/cholesterol-screenings/index.html.

72. Albert L. Siu on behalf of the U.S. Preventive Service Task Force, "Screening
for High Blood Pressure in Adults: U.S. Preventive Services Task Force Rec-
ommendation Statement," *Annals of Internal Medicine* 163, no. 10 (November
2015): 778, doi: www.doi.org/10.7326/M15-2223.

73. "High Blood Pressure: Know Your Risk for High Blood Pressure," Centers
for Disease Control and Prevention, last modified February 24, 2020, www.cdc.
gov/bloodpressure/risk_factors.htm.

74. "How to Spot Skin Cancer," American Cancer Society, last modified April
9, 2020, www.cancer.org/latest-news/how-to-spot-skin-cancer.html.

75. U.S. Preventive Service Task Force, "Screening for Cervical Cancer: Recom-
mendation Statement," *American Family Physician* 99, no. 4 (February 2019):
252B, URL: chrome-extension://oemmndcbldboiebfnladdacbdfmadadm/www.
aafp.org/afp/2019/0215/od1.pdf.

76. "Gynecologic Cancers: What Are the Symptoms?" Centers for Disease
Control and Prevention, last modified August 7, 2019, www.cdc.gov/cancer/
gynecologic/basic_info/symptoms.htm.

77. "Incidence, Prevalence, and Cost of Sexually Transmitted Infections in the
United States," Centers for Disease Control and Prevention, CDC Fact Sheet,

last modified August 29, 2013, npin.cdc.gov/publication/incidence-preva-lence-and-cost-sexually-transmitted-infections-united-states.

78. David Meyers, Tracy Wolff, Kimberly Gregory, Lucy Marion, Virginia Moyer, Heidi Nelson, Diana Petitti, and George F. Sawaya "USPSTF Recom-mendations for STI Screening," *American Family Practice* 77, no. 6 (March 2008): 819, PMID: 18386598.

79. "Incidence, Prevalence, and Cost of Sexually Transmitted Infections in the United States"; Meyers, "USPSTF Recommendations for STI Screening," 819.

80. Meyers, "USPSTF Recommendations for STI Screening," 819.

81. "Incidence, Prevalence, and Cost of Sexually Transmitted Infections in the United States"; Meyers, "USPSTF Recommendations for STI Screening," 819.

Index

vaginal delivery
positions for, 137-140
pushing for, 130-132
vaginal seeding, 141
weight gain, 126
Preterm labor, 127-128, 132,
134-135, 173
Proctalgia fugax, 90
pelvic pain resources for, 185-186
Pudendal nerve:
anatomy, 10-11
neuralgia, 90
pelvic pain resources for, 185-186

R

Rectal splinting:
definition, 16-17
in Rome criteria, 70
with toilet posture, 76-78
see also constipation
Recto-anal contractile reflex (RACR), 64
Recto-anal inhibitory reflex (RAIR), 64
RED-S (Relative energy deficiency in sport), 154-155

S

Sexual assault resources, 184
Sexually transmitted diseases (STD), 153, 156, **172-173**
pelvic pain, contributions to, 89, 91
Smoking cessation resources, 184
Stretching:
for constipation, 73-74
groin, 105
hip, 103-104
low back, 103
pelvic floor muscles for pelvic pain, 100-101
pelvic floor muscles postpartum, 146-147

pelvic floor muscles in pregnancy, 130-131
Substance abuse resources, 180-181

T

Toilet posture, 27, 76-78

U

Urethra caruncle, 157
monitoring, 26
Urinary incontinence, 50-58
in adolescence, 154, 156
insensible, 55-56
in menopause, 157
mixed, 55
overflow, 55-56
pads for, eliminating, 57-58
postpartum, 144
stress, 51-54
urge, 54-55
urgency and frequency, contributing to, 47-50
see also knack
Urinary tract infection, 58-59
cranberry juice and, 44-45

V

Vaginal delivery, 140-141
birthing positions, 137-140
perineal massage, 130-131
pushing, 130-132
recovery, 146-147
Vaginal seeding, 141
Vaginal weights, 22, **118-119**
Vaginismus, 90-91
with other diagnoses, 88, 91
pelvic pain resources for, 185-186
Valsalva:
with bowel movements, 78
definition, 16
hemorrhoids, contributions to, 84

About the Author

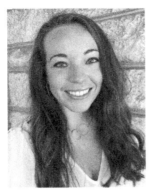

Dr. Megan Rorabeck, DPT, WCS, a board-certified women's health clinical specialist physical therapist, is recognized as a specialist through the American Physical Therapy Association. Dr. Rorabeck founded Between the Hips, LLC, to provide education and empowerment on women's health topics via writing, coaching, and speaking platforms. As a full-time practicing clinician, she helps patients return to living the life they enjoy. She also teaches courses for the Doctorate of Physical Therapy program at her alma mater, Carroll University.

Dr. Rorabeck enjoys camping and fishing, competing in triathlons, reading, and traveling. She loves a good cup of coffee, a beautiful sunset, the smell of the salty ocean, a cool breeze on a hot day, and being surrounded by laughter. Recently, Dr. Rorabeck and her husband, Brian, adopted a shepherd-mix dog, Vortex, who adds a sweet and spunky touch to their lives.

Made in the USA
Monee, IL
04 April 2023